"Spoiler alert: *Cancer as a Love Sto[ry?]* cancer. Author Gail Kauranen Jor[es] cancer, takes on the central failur[e] emotions in health and disease. H[...]  [...] brutally honest story takes the reader through her amazing journey of building new brain connections to enable healing through connection to community, nature, and the divine. Her transformed mindset is focused on new possibilities and self-affirmation. The book offers an abundance of tools, tips, resources, and lessons learned from both western and alternative approaches. Gail points the way forward for anyone interested in a new American dream: life, liberty, and the pursuit of neuroplasticity."

—PHYLLIS STRUPP
Brain training expert and award-winning author of
The Richest of Fare and Better with Age:
The Ultimate Guide to Brain Training

"A high-five to Gail Kauranen Jones for giving us the powerfully compelling chronicle of a wakeup call. She tells it like it is, without pulling her punches, and simultaneously makes it supremely informative, jam-packed with usable links and leads. With grace and grit, she has used her illness for what all illnesses were designed for— to get our attention and reorient us, encouraging us to embrace not only the habits of optimal health, but perhaps the much harder human work of falling back in love with ourselves."

—GREGG LEVOY
New York Times best-selling author of
Callings: Finding and Following an Authentic Life and Vital Signs:
The Nature and Nurture of Passion

"For too long breast cancer has been considered primarily a 'women's issue.' Gail's story will inspire both men and women—especially men who dearly love a woman dealing with the tragic impact of hearing these four life-shattering words: *'You have breast cancer'.*"

—DAVID BRADSHAW
Publisher, myideafactory.net

"Gail Kauranen Jones, a cancer survivor, has written a very compassionate and educational book in which she provides the right combination of medical information and options for personal actions and techniques, all in nontechnical terms, and easily readable language. She provides an 'insiders' view of treatment options, encourages people with cancer to change their past attitudes and beliefs, embrace a new and optimistic future, and live more vibrant lives. Not to be missed are the 'tips' that she offers throughout the book. Her book is a 'must read' for anyone with cancer, anyone who has a family member or a friend with cancer, and for healthcare providers. It will change their lives. Any reader will be inspired."

— DR. ANN WEBSTER
Health psychologist, professor, and former director,
The Mind Body Program for Cancer at
Massachusetts General Hospital

"*Cancer as a Love Story* is open, brave, and has the intellect of a journey well done. It is an invitation to sit with self, allow the inner knowing to surface, then trust it to guide you. Gail's story gives clarity and hope for healing. The book's approach is truly integrative and holistic."

—SHERRY ZUMBRUNNEN, BSN, MN, RN, HNBC
(specializing in working with cancer patients),
Certified yoga instructor, and Reiki master

"When your soul and spirit are touched by God, your body and psyche respond. In turning everything over to God and having strong faith, you open a door for Him to walk in and perform miracles. Whether immediate or progressive, God's healing hand is ready to transform your life. Gail Kauranen Jones has written a book of hope, healing and heart. Just by opening to the first page, Gail shows that she is willing to let light and love into life. Miracles await!"

—SARA BUCKNER O'MEARA
Nobel Peace Prize nominee, renowned spiritual healer,
and leader of The Little Chapel ministry, Paradise Valley, AZ

"In all the years we have been associated professionally and personally, Gail's beautiful spirit has known no bounds when it comes to writing and teaching. Her book, *Cancer as a Love Story,* epitomizes in most exquisite ways her commitment to helping others through sharing her story and the lessons she has learned in life. It is impossible to imagine that her words will not offer deep comfort and life-changing insights to those who read this book."

—DIJANA WINTER, M.Ed.
Psychotherapist, spiritual coach, and teacher

"Gail's book, *Cancer as a Love Story*, shares the truth about healing from the inside out. She skillfully teaches us, with great depth and vulnerability, the emotional release necessary to detox the body of harmful negative toxins. Gail is a true pioneer in teaching us how to use 'energy as medicine' and the latest advances in neuroscience to train the mind to heal the body. I am in awe of her courage, wisdom, and tenacity, to use her healing journey as an empowering and hopeful example for others."

—FLORENCE GAIA, RN, M.Ed.
Holistic nurse and therapist

"Trusting, believing, and following her intuition and proactively changing, Gail Kauranen Jones has done what it takes to truly heal a disease from the inside out. Sharing her intimate journey of transformation, readers can walk with her, learning how to utilize a toolbox of alternative therapies to shift their energy and create the foundation upon which healing takes place. Her valuable insights beautifully parallel key concepts practiced in the ancient and powerful Traditional Chinese Medicine approach, where diseases are seen as imbalances that ultimately begin with an emotion. If one must choose between repression or expression, it is better to choose expression so the energy doesn't manifest internally. An added bonus: Gail's compassionate style of sharing allows the reader to feel a kinship with her and to know they are *not* alone."

—DIANA DAGROSA, MSOM, L.Ac., CAN
Founder/Owner of brightpathwellness.com

"*Cancer as a Love Story* contains a wealth of treasures for people wanting to explore the full spectrum of their healing options after a cancer diagnosis. Gail Kauranen Jones shares straight-up her first-hand experiences with medical modalities from conventional to the fringe, just as a friend might tell you about the good, the bad, and the ugly of her experience. Even more important, she delves into who we need to become in order to allow sustained healing to occur. Curl up with a cup of hot tea and dive in!"

—DR. SHANI FOX, ND
Healing and Hope for Cancer Survivors
www.drshanifox.com

CANCER

as a

Love Story

Developing
the Mindset for *LIVING*

GAIL KAURANEN JONES

Year of the Book
135 Glen Avenue
Glen Rock, PA 17327

ISBN 13: 978-1-945670-55-8
ISBN 10: 1-945670-55-X

This book is in no way a medical prescription of any kind. Rather, it is my story of reinvention from the inside out, prompted by a cancer diagnosis. The book's intention is to share resources of hope and possibility for greater health, which I gleaned from five years of research and participation in a variety of healing approaches.

The core of my healing work included using the latest discoveries in neuroscience, the new field of epigenetics, "energy as medicine," and my faith journey to help train my mind and open to the power of spirit to heal my body.

While traditionally the focus has been primarily on physical healing to move beyond cancer, which was indeed part of my journey, my greatest challenge was courageously facing and releasing emotional toxins that contributed to the stress that may have brought on my cancer diagnosis.

As both a transformational leader and coach, and now a patient, I offer a unique insider glimpse on what it takes to release internal stressors.

Whether one engages in conventional or alternative healing modalities—or a combination of both as I did—it is my belief the underlying emotional causes that contributed to the disease must be addressed for optimal healing potential. Unfortunately, few in our conventional medical paradigms know how to teach this information, and if they do, they are limited by insurance-mandated time constraints in sharing the tools.

Cover Design: Rose Russo, Pathways Graphic Design
www.pathwayslifeasart.com

DEDICATION

To my granddaughter
Leila Elizabeth Maloof

May you (and all children) grow in perfect
health by living from an innate sense of love
and worthiness.

Acknowledgments

"At times our own light goes out and is rekindled by a spark from another person. Each of us has cause to think with deep gratitude of those who have lighted the flame within us." — Albert Schweitzer

Throughout my healing journey, I consistently learned that gratitude is one of the most potent contributors to living a life of joy and well-being. I am blessed that so many people championed me through the five years of bootstrapping this book to completion. Without your help, this "calling" to serve messages of love, worthiness, and hope to those newly diagnosed would not have been fully honored.

This calling, like many of you, arrived quite unexpectedly. It appeared in the middle of the night, when I jumped out of bed after receiving the title of the book. I began writing nonstop for days after initially vowing I would keep my cancer journey private. Callings have a way of nudging you forward in directions you cannot foresee!

So many times, when I ran out of time or money, I wanted to bail on this project. Thanks to the love, encouragement, and practical help from those of you listed below, collectively, this book made it to market. May you each feel part of someone's healing that results from **incorporating some of the tools, techniques, or insights contained within these pages.**

Some contributions overlap with people assisting me within more than one category (and please know I know that, but for simplicity purposes I chose one in which to acknowledge you):

My spiritual mentors and companions:

Dijana Winter

Flo Gaia

Linda Salazar

Marj Elliott

Catherine Russell

Meg Moran

Sara O'Meara

Those who housed me (or gave me space in which to write):

Carrie Hayden

Judy Miller

Sue Rickard

Sharon Hildebrandt

Suzanne Gaker

Barbara J Hopkinson

Those who gave financial support:

Bill Robertson

Beth Scanzani

Wayne Kauranen

Billy Kennerley

Lisa Ackerman and Scott May

Carol Soyster Marshall & Family

Laura Broderick

Rick Sokolow

Cynde Denson

Craig Hopkins

Mike Reed

Sharon Spector

My Arizona team who held me, very tightly at times (thank God), through my reinvention 3,000 miles away from all I knew:

Jess Cullen

Joyce McDonough

Lisa Langaker

Emily Gardner Foppe

Dr. Karla Birkholz

Sharon Winningham and her Love Groups

David Burns

Margaret Swantko

Wayne Benenson

Barbara Jean Gordon

The book team:

Production skills are essential in bringing a book to market, but it was the generosity of spirit that kept the momentum going in working with these next few special people.

My editor, Demi Stevens, of Year of the Book, rightly calls herself a "book whisperer." Her ability to help hone my creativity to "clean closets" (as she calls the foundational process of bringing a book to market) was profound. The organizing of a book is as critical as the writing. Demi was top-notch at pulling diverse pieces collected over five years into a readable manuscript that flows. She provided a breadth of technical skills, intuitive insights, and marketing savvy that kept the book aligned with my larger mission.

My graphic designer, Rose Russo, brought the lovely combination of sophistication and warmth to the branding of my coaching and writing business. Later, she created the book cover and related materials that evolved my practice into a teaching platform of love and worthiness.

Talented author David Bradshaw generously provided his time and editing eyes, offering valuable feedback during the last stretch of this journey. Cyndi Deal, who did the final proofread, was also instrumental in providing emotional and physical support through my early healing journey.

For all of you who believed in me, in whatever capacity you contributed to my journey, I am forever grateful.

CONTENTS

INTRODUCTION

Saying Yes to Life

This is the book I wish my doctors had given me when I was first diagnosed with breast cancer in May 2012. Better yet, I wish I had received it decades earlier. Perhaps, if I knew what I have since learned from five years of my healing journey and ongoing research, I may have been able to prevent the dreadful disease from developing.

Conventional medicine is needed, especially for diagnosis, but unfortunately, the majority of traditional doctors are not equipped to explain or teach the alternative healing methods you will learn about in this book. Rather than being limited by "either/or" thinking, I believe patients must choose the right blend of treatments for themselves based on their mindset and state of health. Let's call it "both/and" thinking.

My goal is simply to provide an insider's look at what some of these other options look and feel like, particularly within the evolving field of "energy as medicine." At the same time, I hope to teach you the healing power of reclaiming your worthiness.

Cancer is a wake-up call, and even when not terminal, can feel like a death—the death of your old self's trauma and drama, and the death of early life conditioning that unknowingly (or subconsciously) allowed more stress into your daily life.

Some see illness as a physical challenge; for me it was an emotional one, to clear all the inner debris that prevented me living from love, so my body could flourish inside a new mindset.

No DNA or physician's report can tell me what I intuitively know about why I got cancer, just as surely as I knew there was something wrong with my mother long before she was officially diagnosed as a schizophrenic. Running on adrenaline most of my life, in the high stress mode of fight-or-flight to override the frightened feelings I ingrained as child, wore my body out. My immune system finally crashed.

Our intuition is wise, and if we quiet ourselves enough to hear the messages of our bodies, we can receive treasures of information about how to heal our ailments. As helpful as they can be in diagnosing, physicians do not have access to our own intuitive wisdom that can be a valuable part of every patient's care package.

I specifically share with you the powerful tools, insights, and techniques I learned to embrace the emotional detox, one of the most overlooked yet necessary parts of the healing process.

A plethora of healing modalities can contribute to your health. My hope is that this book will help you see cancer as a way to create a new love story for yourself. By committing to change your past and embrace a new future, you can live a more fulfilling and vibrant life—before, during, and after a cancer diagnosis.

PART ONE:

RAW BEGINNINGS

NOT ME, PLEASE

The room became eerily cold, as a tray of cookies and coffee were offered to me. The nursing manager assured me everything would be fine.

Like many women with fibrocystic breasts, I had been called back for a repeat mammogram a few times in the past. This year I was asked to stay for an ultrasound and told not to worry, that this extra step is often needed for a closer look beyond what a radiologist can read on the mammogram. Yet there was nothing normal about this extra waiting time, or being escorted down the hall to a private room.

With the intensity of waiting for a big, dark secret to be brought to light, I felt suffocated by the terror of what was to be revealed.

How much longer could I hold in my fright, intuitively knowing something was terribly wrong? Too much sweetness and kindness were being offered to me in this secluded room, in the way one feels pity when they are at a disadvantage or about to be told a loved one has just died.

Soon a perky social worker dressed in funky red glasses and a stoned-faced, gray-haired radiologist appeared. In a flat tone with no warmth or compassion, the radiologist informed me that x-rays revealed what he believed to be a suspicious cancerous tumor on my right breast.

The social worker began asking questions about my children and their ages, and my relationship status. My anxiety levels escalated, as I felt like I was being prepared for last rites and asked whom to notify upon my death. *"Don't bring my kids into this,"* I wanted to yell in that primal, maternal way. *"This is my shock to handle; don't you dare let it touch them."*

In reality, the social worker was only trying to catch a grasp of my family support system. Suddenly, being a single divorced mother felt even more lonely, as there was no other half of a partnership at home to cushion the news, or stand strong to comfort and/or distract my children while I tried to grasp the enormity of the words I'd just heard.

This was worse than any pink slip of termination I ever imagined; this was potential entry into the "pink ribbon" club, for which I never applied to become a member.

Rattled about the possibility of my own physical extinction, I went into defiance. My survival instincts came roaring forth, fighting the doctor's medical evaluation. I would not allow cancer to ever become a reality. It wasn't in my life plan. Maybe if I got angry enough, I could dismiss the words I had just heard.

"Could it be a cyst?" I asked, desperately pleading that the radiologist would change his mind. Looking grimly at me, the doctor said it looked more serious than that.

The tears and terror squelched too long from hours of waiting came gushing forth. I sobbed, "This can't happen to me, I am a single mother with two teenage children. I've already been through enough challenges in my life." This 'Why me?' victim mentality was prompted by excruciating levels of vulnerability at this most raw moment of my life.

I saw briefly a scary picture in my mind of my kids becoming motherless, and not being able to watch them grow into adults. The lovely nurse manager listened as I absorbed the shock of the potential cancer diagnosis. I would need a biopsy to see if the radiologist's suspicions about my lump were true.

Thankfully, a friend who had come to the appointment to support me was there in the waiting room. She took me out for an ice cream. Numb, I knew on that day that any control I thought I had about my life was gone. I could only control my emotions.

THE DAY THE RESULTS CAME IN

On May 4, 2012, the results came in while I was in a business meeting. Stepping outside to take the call, I was told I had breast cancer and more specific results would be forthcoming.

My business partner at the time did her best to distract me, which meant we continued on like nothing happened, meeting with a professional colleague hours later as planned. Talk about denial!

Then, alone at home feeling like I was on a deserted island with no rescue in sight, there was more waiting, more anxiety, and the most intense prayers of my life.

Not yet connected to the spiritual source of comfort I would later engage with on this journey, I kept asking, *"Where is everybody?"* Like the little girl who once felt abandoned by her mom, I got triggered by feelings of acute loneliness and was shamefully afraid to tell anyone of my cowardice.

I was frozen, numb, and in terror. Yet, I could no longer feign feeling stronger than I was in this moment by "sucking it up" as I had in the past. I was vulnerable and needed to find a way to let others know I needed them. Walls of self-protection and ego-driven pride crumbled around me. It had become my time to receive and be inner-directed—a very uncomfortable role reversal from serving as a life coach for others.

My body was exhausted. The game as I knew it was over forever. I would never be the same again. Nothing prepared me for being suspended between the familiar, stoic life I had before and a new one of uncertainties. There was no turning back, no changing the dial, and no redoing of all the stressors that contributed to my hearing those four dreadful words: *You have breast cancer.*

Lying in bed alone at night, I sobbed into my pillow while waiting for the next set of results that would confirm the size and stage of the tumor. This waiting felt like the cruelest penalty ever. I wanted a mommy to hold me, to cuddle in a nurturing chest and be cradled. I also longed for a partner to share this unexpected path, to look into loving, compassionate, and kind eyes and have strong, caring arms hold me. I wanted to melt and be comforted; this was too big to handle alone.

I prayed: *"I am so scared. God, hear my words. My kids need me. Divorce was hard enough on them. I need to live. Please, please, please, keep me alive,"* as I continued to gush tears of release into the pillow night after night.

TIPS

1. Pause, retreat and ground yourself before making any decisions. Turn off your cell phone, stop discussing treatment options with others, and go within to ask for guidance. Center in love versus fear.
2. Trust in your body's innate ability to heal and align with others who hold that possibility for you.
3. Focus on the end result of how you want to be living your life three, five, ten and twenty years from now.
4. Start meditating at least 20 minutes daily.
5. Begin a spiritual practice whether it is going to church, praying, reading the Bible, *A Course in Miracles*, or other consciousness-raising literature or philosophy.

THE HIGH STRESS OF WAITING

Waiting for test results was definitely the highest stress I ever felt.

Unlike when you are waiting to learn if you are pregnant while trying to conceive a child—and anxiously wanting to share the excitement of a new life—standing by to hear if you have cancer is terrifying.

Then, even when you hear the dreaded "C" word, there are many more tests and weeks of waiting for final results. The mammogram showed one image, the biopsy ultrasound another, and the MRI portrayed a third result. Then, upon removal of the lump a few weeks later, another round of pathology tests were run to make a final diagnosis. For me, this was a six-week journey of courage, strength, and vigilance of holding positive thoughts in my mind for the best possible outcome.

Every time the phone rang and I saw the hospital number on my caller ID, I had to ground myself, and pray for grace. Some calls were only to confirm appointments, not reveal test results.

In the waiting time, I made a commitment to deal with cancer holistically, by respecting my mind, body, and spirit, which required significant amounts of additional "unbillable hours" cutting into my income stream.

On days when time felt short, cancer also increasingly felt like a huge inconvenience—an energy-sucking, time-snatching, full-time job on top of my other responsibilities of running a business and mothering.

I now had to spend all my "free" time researching treatment options, participating in alternative care healings to calm my body and mind, and take many, many walks in the serenity of nature to tune into my inner wisdom.

Just as I was learning to protect my mind by carefully focusing on what thoughts were allowed to gain entry, I also became vigilant about my physical body. With the help of a nutritionist, I initiated a new diet plan that eliminated wheat, sugar, and dairy to reduce the possibility of new cancer cells forming.

Distraction was another part of my initial strategy. I was co-operating a blog writing and marketing business to complement my coaching practice. My business partner, who had been through her own share of health challenges, was a genius at keeping me busy and involved in our professional lives. She also was an amazing source of strength and wisdom. In fact, because of our own personal experiences and expertise we focused a niche of our business on health and wellness clients.

To function daily as a mother, friend, and professional when not knowing if you are going to live or die, is a very tough balancing act. Some days I was more short-tempered and frazzled with people than I would have liked. On other days, I felt triumphant, expecting only good news.

I also chose to only tell those people who I knew would be loving and supportive of me during my health challenge, and who could also hold the intention for a positive outcome. I did not want to create any drama around the diagnosis.

TIPS

1. Find ways to distract yourself and stay busy while waiting for test results.

2. Associate with loving, positive people who believe in your good health.

3. Pamper yourself as much as possible, either by doing a favorite activity or taking time just for to be alone with yourself. You and your health are now a priority!

4. Become proactive: choose to educate yourself in ways to stay healthy.

Instead of reading any fear-based information on cancer, I chose to research stories and data about people who gained wonderful insights or went on to create happy lives. The process of waiting taught me that we all have the power to talk in loving and supportive ways to ourselves no matter the outcome.

A week later, the next round of results from the pathology report was given to me at the hospital. The verdict was early-stage breast cancer—good news! Another friend came with me to take notes, as there was so much technical information to take in. We spent four, exhausting hours meeting a team: the surgeon, the oncologist, the radiologist, the nurse practitioner, and the social worker. Surgery to remove the lump was necessary before knowing more details.

Relieved that I was not diagnosed at Stage-II, III or IV—and with great empathy for those who have received an even scarier later-stage diagnosis—the impact of hearing the "C" word cannot be underestimated.

Cancer became a wake-up call to change my entire life—diet, mindset, environments, the people I related with, and the depths of spirituality attained. Whether one chooses to have radiation or chemotherapy, or not, cancer is a change in psyche; that's where healing needs to begin.

Like a child tentatively learning a new activity, I now had to wobble through making friends with that new psyche. First, I had to respect its tenderness and embrace an entirely new identity, chosen based on living from love rather than fear. Part of the reframe included extending to myself new levels of kindness and compassion that I had long before only given to others.

To live, I had to become the priority, which is one of the biggest shifts many who get diagnosed with breast cancer need to make.

Being "centered in self" is not the same as being self-centered, which is self-absorption to the exclusion of others. *(Think of the oxygen mask* *metaphor on a plane: we have to fill ourselves up before we can extend most helpfully to others.)*

After diagnosis, the hospital team—while competent and professional—seemed more like a well-rehearsed sales machine. The radiologist tried to bond with me, and made treatments sound like a routine procedure with minimal side effects, by declaring, *"Six weeks and they would be over."* Nothing in my gut told me it was as simple as that, for I knew friends with cancer whose lives were forever changed by radiation. The radiologist's nonchalant manner was so disconcerting that my intuition prompted me to pause; I didn't trust him. I had to start trusting myself.

Like the process of creating a patchwork quilt, I continued to piece together what felt "right" from all the information I gleaned in my research.

TIPS for dealing with the initial diagnosis

1. Bring a friend or someone else who loves you to every meeting. Support helps a lot. When in a raw, emotional state, it can feel overwhelming to hear all the technical information. Having another to take careful notes to read later relieves some of the stress.

2. Stay as busy as possible during all the time waiting for results. Exercise, meditation, yoga, and other mindful activity helps.

In a vulnerable state upon hearing the "C" word, which some say can even ignite feelings of post-traumatic stress, it is sometimes hard to realize that *cancer is also a big business.*

Even the most gifted doctors who want to give greater attention and concern often have mandated quotas to see so many patients per hour. There's often no time for doctors to provide the nurturing compassion that can heal. I felt like a number—not a person—on a conveyor belt of "system procedures" that began feeling increasingly impersonal.

My support system—where I would be seen, heard, validated, and acknowledged on an emotional, physical, spiritual, and mental level—would need to be found elsewhere. This hospital team could only serve as technicians, not my caring tribe that I would later create. It reminded me of when I mistakenly leaned too heavily (at high billable rates) on my attorney before realizing his job was to gather information and file legal documents, not to emotionally support me in moving beyond my marriage.

Life soon took on a new purpose: to make a conscious effort to do as much emotional and spiritual healing as possible, by blending conventional medical approaches with alternative healing techniques using the latest research in neuroscience, the new field of epigenetics, and "energy as medicine." My intention was to clear my body of any negativity from past stressors or early life conditioning to prepare it to get in a restful state to heal.

The subsequent one-on-one meeting with the social worker felt more genuine, as she helped prepare me to share my diagnosis with my children.

TELLING KIDS "THE C WORD"

As an adult, you are frightened enough through the unknowns of hearing a cancer diagnosis. Imagine telling your kids. Too many children (and some adults) equate cancer with death. Cushioning the sharing of that information is critical. I learned of my diagnosis as my daughter was studying for final exams during her junior year of college. My son was completing his freshman year of high school.

I chose to wait to tell my daughter until she returned home for the summer, and I had more specifics about my treatment plan and could explain in person. Sadly, it was our very first conversation upon her return, not the light mother-daughter lunch I had hoped to share prior to our annual manicure/pedicure summer treat. She already knew I had some tests following a mammogram, and she sensed in my phone voice a few weeks earlier that something was wrong. Like many Internet savvy teenagers, she had already researched cancer to learn of high survival rates.

I told my son immediately, as he knew I had a doctor's appointment and could sense I was dealing with a health issue. Honesty is important. Children sense and know the truth.

I also alerted his guidance counselor, in the event my health would affect him any way at school. In fact, his guidance counselor was the first person outside my inner circle of friends and family to know of my health challenge. I sobbed throughout the entire conversation. Sharing a cancer diagnosis beyond my trusted personal relationships made the diagnosis feel real for the first time. Later that same morning, I called back the counselor who I have known for years and more calmly explained my situation, as well as how raw I felt sharing information which was still scary to me.

The breast clinic's social worker helped me walk through how I would share this information with a 15-year-old boy, who I am sure wanted nothing to do with talking about breasts with his mother—never mind the fear of his mom having a life-threatening disease.

She suggested I approach my conversation from a more educational manner, discussing how preventative care is so important. After explaining to my son my diagnosis, following a routine mammogram, he responded, "I see this as just a speed bump in the road of life." I laughed, and later that evening shed a very tender tear.

TIPS

1. Center in yourself, absorbing the news of your diagnosis, before sharing with your children. Then, try to see how they will perceive the information from their age and gender. Select a calm time to share, when they are not in the midst of something very important or challenging to them.

2. Remember (especially if you are a single parent where bonds can be more intense), your children are your kids, not your caretakers. Although you may warrant or be appreciative of extra levels of compassion, you cannot expect your children to do the heavy emotional lifting. Let your kids be kids.

3. Release your fears and anxieties by finding a support system, whether it is a good friend or a professional counselor.

SECOND OPINIONS

I researched my surgeon prior to meeting her and trusted my gut when she first consulted with me. Warm, kind, and clearly confident, she also listened non-judgmentally to my concerns and ideas, including the alternative healings I had undertaken. She even repeated an ultrasound at my request. Her support was clearly evident, as was her level of competence and expertise as she discussed with me how many surgeries she routinely performs.

Upon learning from pathology results that I would need a lumpectomy and one or more sentinel nodes removed, I chose to get a second opinion. Other experts' views can be helpful, but they can also lead to confusion if the recommended treatments are different. *Who needs more confusion?* I initially wondered. The thought of repeating the lengthy consultation process seemed draining and scary. Then, my inner voice urged me (and was validated by friends who were great sounding boards) to move forward with no regrets, knowing I had researched my health options as thoroughly as possible.

As it turned out, I did not need to attend lengthy meetings with a new team. I had my medical records sent via fax. This next surgeon, who was older and had several years more experience working with nationally known breast cancer and women's health doctors, confirmed the recommended surgeries. She also suggested that I request only one sentinel node be taken if possible, and alerted me to a test to determine chance of breast cancer recurrence. Since my first surgeon had already discussed that option with me, it confirmed and solidified my original relationship.

After that second consult, I called the first surgeon with questions, which she promptly and gladly answered. No offense was taken because I had sought a second opinion, which to me further confirmed my gut instinct that she was the right surgeon for me.

Later in the process, when choosing follow-up treatments, these are some good questions I learned to ask my surgeon and other members of the health care team:

1. How many people have you cured?
2. What's the risk?
3. What if I do nothing at all?
4. Would you recommend this same treatment to your spouse or someone you loved?

Choosing a breast surgeon is selecting a doctor you will be in relationship with the rest of your life, as your health will be continually monitored by him or her.

Liking the style, and respecting the expertise of the doctor who will support you, can make your ongoing care a positive and engaging team effort.

TIPS

1. Being proactive about your health empowers you. Choosing to get a second opinion is an option worth exploring, if you have the tiniest inkling that you may regret not doing so.

2. View your surgeon as a partner in your lifelong care, and discern at a gut level and through research who feels right for you.

CIRCLES OF SUPPORT—
ASKING FOR HELP

Until my cancer diagnosis, I had done much in my life physically alone—from raising two children as a single parent and the tasks of managing a home, to running two businesses solo. Being super-responsible was my standard mode of operation. I was someone everyone else could lean on. Yet, I often felt excruciatingly lonely.

Growing an inner circle of women friends—"sisters," spiritual mentors, and guides—helped counter those sad feelings and provide the support and feedback I had given many others in my work as a life coach.

With the surgery challenge ahead, and all the fear I had to push through to stay in a place of calm and self-love, I knew I needed these kind people more than ever. Asking for help—as vulnerable as it felt to do so—became a priority.

Slowly, I put together a list of my confidantes and their contact information. I sent them updates of my health status and each friend stepped up to the plate in unique ways. Some came to doctor appointments with me. Others gifted me massages, alternative healing sessions, and pampering manicure/pedicures. A few did grocery shopping or delivered meals. One girlfriend stayed with me two nights after surgery, taking full charge of my health by cooking nutritious meals. Another took me out to dinner six weeks after recovery, as a celebration of new levels of health. Flowers, cards, and email notes sustained me during some of the darker moments.

The hardest time again, like when I was first diagnosed, was alone in bed at night, longing to be held tenderly to ward off scary thoughts about my longevity. What I did not initially realize was that more than just cancerous breast tissue needed to be excised.

I did not just have a small tumor removed; I released a lifestyle that no longer served me.

TIPS

1. This online meal planner, which my friend Linda Salazar initiated using on my behalf, was a godsend. It enables you, the patient, to select what types of foods best serve your family's needs and taste buds. Friends and other helpers can then log in and choose which days they can provide a related meal: www.lotsahelpinghands.com.

2. Delegate and allow yourself to receive support. Not only is accepting help necessary to give your body time to rest so it can heal faster, but it deepens your connection to one another. Genuine love involves both giving and receiving. Balance the scales by accepting nurturance and support.

3. Take time to observe love and care in the simplest of moments (like when someone brings fresh produce from their vegetable garden).

4. Acknowledge the many diverse ways others show their support for you. (Read *The Five Languages of Love* to learn different styles.) Accept that you are worthy of such care and appreciate those who provide it.

PREPARING FOR SURGERY

Acquiring a Calm State

One month after my initial diagnosis, I was scheduled for surgery, which entailed a lumpectomy and removal of one sentinel node. Many synchronicities led me to the right healers and kept me on the alternative healing path, teaching me skills I now share with clients.

Many times, these connections seemed like "divine intervention," appearing just as I needed the next step of healing.

For instance, my friend, Beth Scanzani, gifted me a session with Peggy Huddleston, an ordained minister who offers healing work at Boston hospitals (www.healfaster.com). Huddleston calmly listened to the stressful events of my previous three years that led me to feeling I had been living on the edge of a cliff—tested financially, emotionally, mentally, and spiritually.

Like Huddleston, my second opinion breast surgeon also said she increasingly noticed that the three years prior to a breast cancer diagnosis were often very stressful years for a patient. Years later, I came to understand better why acupuncturist and Traditional Chinese Medicine (TCM) practitioner Diana DaGrosa urges those at the onset of stress (before an illness appears) to seek treatments that balance and align the body, mind, and spirit.

Huddleston's goal was to initiate a state of calm, which would enable me to better handle surgery and heal faster afterward. Through a guided meditation, she created scenes for my mind to embrace the "end results" I wanted to achieve. Through Huddleston's soft words, I taught my mind to expect a successful surgery and quick recovery. I also focused on reminding my cells of their natural ability to be healthy.

During high levels of stress, outside perspective is enormously helpful to remain grounded in strength. How we communicate with our bodies greatly impacts our health, as I continued to learn. Accepting help, learning to receive, and do for myself what I do for my clients, continued to be a huge part of my healing journey.

Huddleston also reminded me I could return to the calm inner mindset I created whenever feeling stressed by recalling that end result.

In conjunction with private sessions, I also used her book, *Prepare for Surgery, Heal Faster: A Guide of Mind-Body Techniques,* along with guided meditation recordings which I listened to twice a day prior to surgery (and continued to use afterwards to remind my cells of their natural ability to be healthy).

During the week prior to surgery, I took several long, blissful walks on Crane Beach in Ipswich, Massachusetts— the calm, restful place I had envisioned during my meditations. Touched by nature and feeling connected to God, I felt an inner joy, blessed to be alive.

TIPS

1. Prepare for surgery by getting yourself in a calm state to accelerate healing. Meditate, go to yoga, or find moments during the day to be still.

2. Create an inner vision board or mindset of a successful surgery and your healing afterwards.

3. Talk to your body, and remind your cells of their ability to become or stay healthy.

4. Get a massage the night before surgery to relax your body and experience the healing power of touch.

I also did the following journal exercise that I had used before with my coaching clients and that Huddleston also recommended:

I wrote to my diseased body part (my right breast), and asked what it had to teach me. After sitting in quiet for at least 20 minutes, the answer came to me:

"Stop running. Stop living in fear. Those days are over, of running in fear from a schizophrenic mother. It's time to slow down and live from love."

Looking back, despite all my accomplishments, I lived most of life in fight-or-flight mode, first as a young girl desperately trying to survive in a chaotic home, then in later years caretaking elderly parents with my brother while juggling the needs of two young children. Post divorce—single parenting and juggling a myriad of jobs, while facing huge financial struggles during the recession while I had a child in college—I kept running. When I wasn't running, I was always thinking in the terrifying fight-or-flight of basic survival needs, even after spending 30 years consciously healing my childhood and later my marriage wounds.

To heal my body this time, versus my psyche from all the years of inner work, I had to stop and rest. In fact, I wish every doctor upon giving a potential cancer diagnosis would advise patients the same. Better yet, the smart physician might order a patient to take a three-week or longer vacation if there is no urgency to treatment. Being rushed off to lab appointments and meetings with medical teams can create added fear that could result in hasty decisions. Making choices of potentially life-altering consequences while in a high state of anxiety that can be equivalent to post-traumatic stress after hearing a cancer diagnosis, felt unwise to me.

As Dr. Ann Webster, once director of The Mind Body Program for Cancer offered by the Benson-Henry Institute for Mind Body Medicine at Massachusetts General Hospital, which I attended (detailed later in this book) says, **"Healing does not happen when we are racing about."**

The evening prior to surgery I had a massage, which enabled me to sleep soundly and with no need for the anti-anxiety drugs offered to me. Being gently touched and held in comfort prior to surgery felt so loving and reminded me of my body's ability to remain calm. I highly recommend massage to anyone entering surgery as a way to honor the body.

The day of surgery, I awoke peaceful, centered, and ready to be released of cancer from my body (and all "the stories" around the stressors I had been experiencing for years beforehand). Instead of focusing on fear of the unknown ahead, I embraced the love of friends, and their phone calls beforehand. At Huddleston's suggestion, I asked all those who cared about me to hold me in "a pink blanket of love" a half-hour before my surgery was scheduled. I requested the anesthesiologist read statements while I was unconscious (which is when the mind is most receptive) of my desired end-results and beliefs about my renewed health that I had created with Huddleston.

Upon waking from a successful surgery, I needed only one painkiller that evening and thereafter never opened the prescribed bottle.

DAY SURGERY

A Procedure, Not a Healing

With "day surgery" I was fortunate to be able to return home and sleep in my own bed the same evening, with loved ones greeting me upon my arrival. Yet, because family and friends do not visit in the hospital while the healing continues, the extent of the loving support that may be needed afterwards is not fully understood.

To some, it seemed to appear as though I just had a tooth pulled— I went to the hospital, had the lump removed, and it was all over. However, physically and emotionally, breast surgery is just the beginning of a new life journey, which will involve continual check-ups and monitoring, tests, and for some, additional treatment including radiation, chemotherapy, or more surgery. Emotionally, it may require help dealing with Post-Traumatic Stress Disorder (PTSD) and overcoming fear of recurrence, as detailed later in this book.

Surgery was just a procedure. The real shift was in facing mortality, and many "life-in-review" and "dark night of the soul" moments. Like grieving the death of a loved one, there were emotional mood swings—from elation at being alive to the terror of how to go forward with a new mindset to sustain greater health.

The hours at the hospital were more painful and exhausting than I imagined, particularly the pre-op procedure of placing a wire in my breast so the dye to locate lymph nodes could be traced. After having an IV placed in my arm upstairs in the pre-op room, and being told the worst of the pain was over, I was not physically or emotionally prepared for the next step.

I was brought downstairs in a wheelchair to the mammography room—wearing only a hospital johnny. Everything suddenly felt very clinical and cold. With my breast placed on the machine, tears started streaming down my face.

Two hurtful tries later, the wire was successfully placed in my breast. As much as I appreciated the need for technical accuracy so the surgeon could properly locate what she needed to see, this part of the day felt shockingly invasive. It was then I longed for painkillers or sedation, which I was told were not allowed during this procedure. However, from that point on, I would feel no more physical pain.

Wheeled back upstairs, I met with the anesthesiologist, who reviewed my end-result meditative statements (created before with Huddleston) that she would later read as I was going under sedation.

TIPS for Day-After-Surgery Help

1. Educate those who will love and care for you that you need their help, support and understanding beyond the immediate hours following your return home from surgery. Not only has your body been altered but your psyche is changing too.

2. Be sure to have someone stay with you at least two, preferably three nights post "day surgery." Then, be sure someone stops by once a day thereafter to physically check in on you.

My surgeon also checked in on me. Seeing her in scrubs with her hair pulled back under a cap caught me slightly off-guard since I had only seen her fashionably dressed as an accomplished, compassionate woman during our prior office visits. Although the stakes were higher on surgery day, I was comforted by her warm, calm, and reassuring direct presence. I saw her in that moment as a competent doctor clearly in charge and confident.

Moments later I was sedated, and in what seemed like a split second, I was waking up greeted by my dear friend, Meg. She shared the good news of a successful surgery with clear margins, and that only one lymph node had needed to be removed.

Packing up to go home, I accepted one painkiller. I felt so nauseous on the ride home that I almost asked Meg to pull over.

Entering my home, I was groggy and tired. Another friend had come to cook and stay with me for the weekend. My daughter helped me undress for bed, and we shared a laugh over my calling a baby "a cute pudgeball" through my drug-induced and somewhat silly and relaxed state.

During the weekend, I overextended myself, thinking because it had been "only day surgery" that I could venture out 48 hours later as okayed by my medical team. Mistakenly, I attended a friend's small concert. Another friend drove, but walking back to the car, I felt like I was going to keel over. My body was clearly weaker than I thought and I was still emotionally vulnerable.

Looking back, I wish I had given myself a full week of bed rest, simply to read and nurture myself, for I now understand more clearly how important relaxation is to healing. I also wish I had not minimized what occurred, that I had better articulated the vulnerability to those around me of my body being traumatized by a surgical procedure. I needed tender, loving care and the understanding that I had just stepped into a new life journey.

As with all transitions, there would be some shaky moments ahead. Day surgery is a procedure that may last only a few hours, but the healing is ongoing. Integrating a new diet and lifestyle, and discovering the forthcoming version of a new "me" had yet to begin.

A DARK DAY

Post-Surgery Blues

The fifth day after surgery was one of the darkest of my life. With torrential rains outside, I felt an intense gloominess as I wandered around my home, alone, lost and shaky. At one point during this stormy day, I thought I would faint from weakness at doing too much, too quickly after surgery.

Slowing down became critical, and even years afterward, pacing my life is still important. We heal and thrive best in life from a restful and peaceful state. Pausing to reflect in solitude also helps create new outcomes for the life desired beyond cancer. Yet, initially, in stopping from moving about so much, excruciating loneliness set in—similar to the time after a funeral when everyone has left and you are alone with your grief.

Everything happened so fast between my diagnosis on May 4 and surgery on June 1 that my psyche had not quite taken in all I had been through. On this dreary day, I realized, maybe for the first time, that I had a cancerous tumor removed from my body, which has been permanently altered. Up until this point, I was feeling blessed that the tumor was caught and removed early.

Then, a new "reality" set in. I had medical bills to pay, new support systems to find which honored my approach to healing, and as a single woman dating, I would have to find the right time and place to share sensitive medical information. Talk about testing a man's staying power!

As I absorbed the enormity of the recent changes, I continued to long for something familiar and safe, a shoulder to lean on, and a feeling that "someone had my back." Old childhood abandonment wounds reared again, and I felt terrifyingly isolated, not sure anyone knew how scared or lonely I was.

Even with a strong support network of friends and counselors, no one could take away the pain of this hurtful and vulnerable day. My body was not ready to live the active lifestyle I craved and my mind was just beginning to understand I was undergoing a personal transformation. In the process, I had to grieve the old way of being to allow for the new me who would emerge.

TIPS to shift mindset upon hearing a diagnosis

1. Change your behavior and eliminate worry by focusing on the present moment while in conversation, walking, eating, listening, or bathing/showering. Appreciate that "being" is healthier than all the doing. According to information shared at The Mind Body Program for Cancer at Massachusetts General Hospital (MGH), 40 percent of waking time is about the *past*, which is a waste of time, and 50 percent is worrying about the future and "what ifs." Maybe on a good day, 10 percent of present time is in the now. Spend more time just BEING. You can plan, which is not the same as worrying. "Jumping to conclusions is not exercise," just all made up information, as teasingly shared at MGH.

2. Get out of isolation and build rich friendships: a 2006 breast cancer study shared at MGH found that women without close friends were four times as likely to die from the disease as women with 10 or more friends. And notably, proximity and the amount of contact with a friend weren't associated with survival—just having friends was protective.

3. You need to embrace the unknown—your psyche has been changed forever once you get a diagnosis. To create a new mindset for living, it helps to give yourself permission to stay for long periods in the unknown.

CLAIMING YOUR FEMININITY POST-SURGERY

The bandage came off a few days after surgery.

Seeing the new scar on my right breast and under my tennis-playing right arm where the sentinel lymph node was removed, I cried quietly in the bathroom. My womanly body was now different.

My surgeon had told me she would make the scars as cosmetically pleasing as possible, but removing the cancer was her first priority. She succeeded in both. The slash mark across my breast did not show when wearing a low-cut blouse or dress.

Accepting and loving my post-surgery body was an empowering choice for me. Like the wrinkles on my now 60-something face, these scars tell a story—both an old and new one. I am a woman of great courage who has endured much adversity. I did not just have a cancerous tumor removed. I was finding a new discipline within to commit to living a healthy lifestyle, in mind, body, and spirit.

The new story of the remaining scars is that they serve as a daily reminder to love and nurture myself first before genuinely extending to others, feed my body healthy foods, and forgive myself and those who have hurt me.

As a result of this increased focus on self-love, I feel more feminine and sexy than ever. One month after surgery, I wore a low-cut, short black knit sundress to a friend's 60th birthday celebration at her beach house. Many people complimented me on my attire.

Yet, my contentment was not about my bold choice to wear that dress instead of the shorts and tee-shirt I would normally choose.

My peace and happiness came from knowing I had been given a second chance and had chosen to live in a new, more feminine way.

Standing on the deck overlooking the ocean, breathing in the day, I felt calm and poised, trusting in the new woman emerging. Gently I embraced her, and the imperfections that add to her uniqueness.

TIPS

1. Choose to love and accept your post-surgery body, and focus on how it serves you now versus how it may look different (and it's OK and perfectly normal first to grieve any losses you feel).

2. Give permission to express yourself in new feminine ways, either through a wardrobe selection or a way of being.

MISERY DOESN'T LOVE COMPANY— AT LEAST NOT ITS OWN

If you told me, "Junk Food Jill" of earlier years, that I'd be eating spinach and avocado salad with no dressing for lunch, I'd say: "No way... that's no fun." Then, I became a statistic as the one in eight women who are diagnosed with breast cancer.

Choosing to confront the health challenge head-on with a radical overhaul of my diet, I gave up wheat, sugar, and dairy—foods my naturopathic doctor believes add toxins to the body and attract cancer cells.

Like the time I quit smoking 34 years ago, in alleviating these food choices, I experienced withdrawal symptoms of feeling cranky, unbearably frustrated, miserable, and sad.

Plus, changing my diet was the first evidence that I had lost the freedom to do whatever I wanted, when I wanted to do it. Eating was no longer an entertaining joy; it was now a discipline I had to learn. These new restrictions caused much grief, as I let go of many of my spontaneous ways. Fine, gourmet foods were now replaced by "greens."

Grateful to be alive—and to be given a second chance at living more healthily—I became dismayed that this new lifestyle choice was so difficult. I struggled with cravings for sweets and carbohydrates, especially chocolate, ice cream, pasta, and great European hearth bread.

One day after walking the beach, a girlfriend took me out to lunch. Eating a veggie burger on lettuce, without a bun, I felt cheated and deprived. I wanted to indulge in a sandwich wrap, but could not eat the bread with which it was made.

"If it were me, I would do the radiation so I could eat what I want," she joked. Sometimes, I still think radiation and Tamoxifen—the gold plan of conventional medicine—would have been easier, at least short-term. Yet, my intuition insisted I try the radical diet changes before exploring those options.

I had not yet acquired the knowledge of food and cooking techniques that would broaden my cuisine choices. So, I stuck with the basic requirements of protein—preferably every two hours—and lots of fruits and vegetables. Bored with my morning egg, I often wanted to run to the downtown Main Street Market and inhale one of the fresh baked morning glory muffins.

It took discipline, focus, and pushing through a lot of resistance to change to eat in this new manner. Grumpily, I stayed committed to this healthy-eating lifestyle, eventually able to withstand my own company again.

MEETING AND EXPRESSING
"THE BITCH" IN ME

"Real liberation comes not from glossing over or repressing painful states of feeling, but only from experiencing them to the full."

—Carl Jung

During my first MRI to get a clearer image of my cancerous lump prior to surgery, I asked the nurse, who was a 14-year-cancer survivor, if cancer had changed her life in any way. She responded that yes it had in two significant ways for the better. First, she slowed down and became much clearer about her priorities. Second, she learned to speak her mind immediately if something upset her, and she no longer holds onto grudges.

Many people told me upon hearing of my breast cancer that the diagnosis was a message to slow down. Pacing myself is not easy as a high energy person who falls under the Leo astrological sign. I have since learned to take breaks during the day, preferably half-hour stretches, to nurture myself with quiet, rest, and the simple wonders of being. Now much more attuned to the needs of my body, mind, and soul, I also consciously attempt to walk and talk slower. In the past, my speech has been rapid, especially when I got excited or passionate about a topic.

The more significant change is speaking my mind as events occur, not months or years later. One day, a male friend asked if there was anything he could do to help. I said, "Sure, can you help pick up my new grill and deliver it in your van to my house, since it won't fit in my car?" His response was, "I'm sure your son can help you handle that."

Stunned, I replied, "You offered help, but just declined my request." I turned and walked away.

Speaking my mind has felt "bitchy" because I used to relish being "good" and felt appreciated for being "nice." I enjoy my sweet and tender sides, which seem to shine best during vulnerable moments.

Confronting mortality head-on made me more aware that living authentically adds value to every moment. I understand now what that MRI nurse meant when she said she no longer holds things in. Yet, I believe we shouldn't hold onto grievances once they have been expressed, either.

The next time I met my male friend while walking the beach, I was friendly. His deference to help with the grill was an isolated incident. I let it go, and was glad I had voiced my disappointment in the moment.

The "bitch" has appeared many times since, when someone does not follow through on a promise, lies about a fact or circumstance, refuses to hear or see me in their presence, projects their own wounds onto me, or consistently shows up late or disrespects me in other ways.

Beyond assertiveness, I see this more vocal part of me as a protector of my health. I am no longer willing to silence her to please another, or make someone look or feel good when they have misjudged, wronged or been inconsiderate of me.

Yet, I take another step after articulating my feelings. I try "to let it go, and let it flow" by forgiving and blessing the person who has upset me so the angst does not remain in my body.

TIPS

1. Self-love means being authentic and expressing our true feelings appropriately.

2. Integrating our innate wholeness extends beyond being "good." We all have light and dark sides, and many emotions. It is okay to own all of them.

LEARNING TO SAY "NO"

Louise Hay, who was founder of Hay House Publishing, noticed a consistent pattern in women suffering from breast cancer—a tremendous inability to say "no." In her book, *Empowering Women: Every Woman's Guide to Successful Living*, she suggested being raised by parents who used guilt or manipulation for discipline is one possible reason women acquiesce so easily and become people-pleasers.

She further claimed that these women's bodies get exhausted as they become surrounded by those who are constantly asking them to do more than they can comfortably do. Straining themselves for others, people-pleasing women say "yes" to demands they really don't want to do. Often, they keep giving until there is no more nourishment left in them to give.

Hay recommended this affirmation as way to change people-pleasing behavior:

"When I say no to you, I am saying yes to me."

"By the time you have said 'No' to the person three times, he/she will realize that you have become a different person and will stop asking you," she advised.

Dr. Judith Orloff, author of *The Empath's Survival Guide*, said during her book tour: "No" is the end of the sentence. Excuses or defenses are not needed when we decline a request.

Learning to say "no" builds self-respect. By loving ourselves more, we become increasingly open to the love we receive from others.

ONE WITH THE BALL (& LIFE) AGAIN

Playing tennis one night, outside on a late summer evening on a lighted court, I connected to the ball in the same way I had prior to my lumpectomy three months earlier—feeling one with it and my joy of life. Beyond the athletic gains, I noticed that the terror, angst, and depression I had lived through all summer had dissipated. The "old me," who was happy, friendly, and competitive on a tennis court was back.

"You're playing great and haven't lost any of your skill," said a male friend whom I asked to practice alone with me before I started playing socially with groups of people.

Upon first hearing my cancer diagnosis on my right breast—and facing so many unknowns—I was unsure if I would ever be able to raise my arm again to play my favorite sport. Still, without any sensory feeling under my right arm where a lymph node was removed, I did not know if my ability to serve a tennis ball would be limited.

Fortunately, playing tennis again came as naturally to me as getting back on a bike. Engaging in athletics reminds me how lucky I am to have full use of my body. More importantly, doing things I used to do before my cancer diagnosis brings my life back to a feeling of normalcy, even though I know I have been changed emotionally, physically, and spiritually forever.

> ## TIPS
>
> 1. Pace yourself and take baby steps as you test the abilities of your body. *The Kaizen Way... One Small Step Can Change Your Life*, by Robert Maurer, Ph.D., is an excellent resource for anyone embracing positive and sustainable change.
>
> 2. Ask for the gentle support of others.

LYMPHEDEMA

A lifelong risk post cancer

According to the Mayo Clinic, lymphedema is the swelling that occurs in one of your arms or legs. Although it tends to affect only one appendage, sometimes both arms or legs may swell.

Lymphedema is caused by a blockage in the lymphatic system, an important part of your immune and circulatory systems. This blockage prevents lymph fluid from draining well, and as it builds up, the swelling continues. It is most commonly caused by the removal of, or damage to lymph nodes as part of cancer treatment.

There is no cure for lymphedema, but it can be controlled through diligent care of your affected limb.

After my lumpectomy I was incorrectly told I could return to normal activity whenever it felt "right." A month or so later, I tried to resume lifting weights, only to feel shooting pain through my right breast, where my cancerous tumor had been removed.

I was working part-time at a health club, and fortunately, had a great personal trainer who handed me information on lymphedema. It was the first time anyone warned me I had to be cautious about the amount of pressure or weight applied to that healing quadrant of my body.

In fact, not one of my doctors—whether conventional or naturopathic—had ever cautioned me about doing heavy lifting on the same side as my surgery, or even asked if they should draw blood from my left arm instead of the right.

Finally an oncology-based massage therapist was able to educate me on the specific facts about cancer-related lymphedema. (Check out breastcancer.org for more information.) Most importantly, she stressed that anyone who has had even one lymph node removed is at a lifetime risk for lymphedema. Specifically, research show 5 to 40 percent of women experience lymphedema after lymph node dissection. Removing fewer nodes may reduce the risk.

Here's what she shared:

- No blood or needle work should be done to the arm where a lymph node has been removed.
- Avoid high heat, especially in steam rooms, saunas, and hot tubs, which can trigger it.
- Sunburns and insect bites can contribute to it.
- Avoid any aggressive joint movement to that quadrant.
- No overexertion—five-pound weight limit on that arm. Be sure also not to carry heavy handbags or luggage on the side where a lymph node was removed.
- Wear no restrictive clothing in that area.
- No increased circulation with heat, ice, friction, and joint movement.
- Injury, cuts, pressure, overstretching, overuse, and infection also trigger lymphedema.

Oncology-based massage is something I now advise all cancer patients to consider. This treatment differs from regular massage in that it uses only light pressure to the quadrant where surgery was performed, and strokes go down and across the back of that area instead of using upward motions.

Massage can be therapeutic for healing and great for relaxation. However, be sure your therapist is properly trained and that neither the massage table (or stones if used as part of the treatment) are not too hot.

Additional resources:
lymphnet.org, www.TracyWalton.com

Lymphedema symptoms

- Swelling of part of (or the entire) arm or leg, including fingers or toes.
- A feeling of heaviness or tightness in the arm or leg.
- Restricted range of motion in arm or leg.
- Aching or discomfort in arm or leg.
- Recurring infections in affected limb.
- Hardening and thickening of the skin on arm or leg.

The swelling caused by lymphedema ranges from mild, hardly noticeable changes, to extreme swelling that can make limb use impossible. If your lymphedema is caused by cancer treatment, you may not notice any swelling until months or years after treatment.

THE ROUGH SEAS OF LIFE
KEEP US ENGAGED

Sailing for the first time ever—amidst sudden, pre-storm conditions no less—I laughed as I got repeatedly splashed by waves from rough waters. Despite occasionally murmuring "shit" when the boat tipped too high up on one side, I felt incredibly safe with my friend, who easily maneuvered the boat in less than ideal conditions.

At least the water is warm if we flip over, I thought to myself, before comprehending that my companion, a former Boy Scout who grew up sailing, was fully in control.

Feeling safe with a strong and intelligent adult taking charge was a gift after several months of living on the edge of healthcare challenges. I also felt a huge sense of relief from being able to lean into someone else's competence after making so many tough decisions and life choices.

At the same time, after staring more closely at my own mortality, the importance of embracing life as an adventure felt paramount. I chose to see these less than calm waters as a moment to stay fully engaged. My now wet, wind-blown hair, pants plastered to my body like a wet tee-shirt contest, and mascara dripping from my eyelids felt surprisingly freeing—like a victory over

TIPS

1. Excuse the pun, but not all of life is smooth sailing. Adjust your attitude to meet the varied conditions of the day. Find the silver lining.

2. Leaning is not co-dependency. Sometimes, it is darn-right nurturing to be with a person who can take charge and be strong for you, particularly after you have just been physically, emotionally, mentally, and spiritually tested through an illness or disease.

the more packaged, perfect-looking demeanor I wore in the past when I erroneously believed I could control my life.

Cancer, like unexpectedly rough waters, taught me to make the best of the scary situations before me. Attitude is everything.

A LIFE SENTENCE

I knew my life would change forever as soon as I heard the words I had breast cancer. I also knew I had the power to reframe those diagnostic words to empower instead of scare me. Rather than search the web and medical books, I opted first to create my own meaning for this next chapter of my life. I immediately dubbed the diagnosis "a life sentence."

Intuitively, I knew a positive attitude and a restful, calm state would be crucial to healing and bringing my body back to optimal levels of health. There were many moments of fear and panic as I awaited each set of test results, but planning time for solitude helped.

I chose to see this red flag or temporary detour in my plans as a sign to redirect my life, even though I was not sure how it would unfold. Adamant that it was just a sidestep, I told friends, "I will never be the breast cancer blogger. This part of my life won't be shared biweekly with my readers."

Later, it became clear that writing is in my bones, and I was meant to share—not just about cancer, but about loving ourselves through the midst of a health challenge versus scaring ourselves. Yet I needed to live in this new mindset before I could share it with others.

Increasingly, I fine-tuned my discernment skills while also detaching more and "letting go"—another paradoxical challenge of taking charge versus trusting and having faith. The greatest shift was in reclaiming my worthiness through self-love.

Part of the ways I learned to love myself, which you can employ too, are to:

- Become an educated, proactive consumer. Information is power. Continually research, ask questions, get second opinions, then go within to access your own wisdom, taking charge, trusting, and having faith.
- Work with a nutritionist to create a healthy diet and stay accountable as you change your eating habits and food choices.
- Make yourself a priority. An investment in your health is the best gift you can give yourself, your children and others you love.
- Exercise 30 minutes daily. I was repeatedly taught that "Cancer cells cannot survive/thrive in a well-oxygenated body."
- Create meditative time, to slow your pace and take in the moments of the day. Trees really do look greener, food tastes better, and the love and kindness of friends feels deeper when you are fully present.
- Associate with people who are kind, positive, and supportive and who will be gentle with you in vulnerable moments. I know I hear information or feedback better when it is delivered with compassion, acceptance, and empathy, versus harshness or judgment. I learned that I can listen to others whose communication styles differ, but I do not have to hire them as an integral part of my team.

Questions for Healing

1. How do I heal this tumor, life distraction, or curveball? What can I do, be, think or feel? Is there a need—physical, mental, emotional, or spiritual—I am not attending to that needs to be addressed now?

2. How does renewed health look and feel in my body? Visualize that answer consistently 3-8 minutes a day.

3. How can I empower myself today to live more vibrantly? (Is there an action step I can take within the next 24 hours to raise my energy level?)

THE HOLIDAY CRASH

Holidays often ignite "a-year-in-review" type of reflection, which for me resulted in a dark night of the soul. Focused intently on loving myself better and surrounding myself with positive people, I was taken aback by the holiday blues, which suddenly emerged.

Grateful to be alive, I thought I would enjoy celebrating. Instead, I suffered intense moments of loneliness and apathy, wondering how I had come to that point in my life as a single mother about to face the initial pangs of an empty nest alone as a cancer survivor.

The story I had scripted for myself did not entail health challenges, nor did it include living without a family to back me up emotionally on top of unexpected financial challenges set off by the recession. The initial wretchedness of my early childhood abandonment re-awoke. Tears gushed unexpectedly to new and old friends.

"You're learning you're not perfect," a wise friend encouragingly suggested. I have intuitively known that seeing my "flaws" was one of the messier lessons of cancer, where my guard of bravado would be knocked to the ground. Other friends also have told me that I seldom show my vulnerability—and instead project an image of togetherness.

That holiday, I showed my despair, even to a client, who lovingly held me in the sacredness of compassion. Releasing the loneliness and terror of the cancer diagnosis is a process, which increasingly makes room for expanded feelings of joy and gratitude for second chances.

In talking with other cancer survivors, I learned it is common after running on adrenaline the first six months, the reality of the trauma then sets in. For me, that time fell at the holidays. In brief flashes, I wondered if that would be my last Christmas.

Then I immediately squelched those fear-based thoughts. Still, I chose to give my children a few meaningful books as presents, to share wisdom I hoped they would absorb and also pass on to their children.

I also mindfully observed my kids and those I cared about, being sure to take in the essence of those around me. I was blessed to receive the healing touch of affection from a man I had been dating, feeling cradled in comfort, care, and laughter after a shocking year.

Circles expanded and deepened when I let go of judgments and stopped looking at the "flaws" of others, and focused on looking for what was "right" about each person or situation. All life has adversity and learning "to bless the mess" relieves the stress, according to Dr. Ann Webster of The Mind Body Program for Cancer.

Post holidays, I indulged in more downtime to rest, integrate the ways I have changed, and set new intentions. Having more fun and a greater appreciation for simple times—like a walk in the woods, sitting by a fire watching a Patriots football game on TV, and spending quality time with friends and loved ones—jumped to the top of the list.

Living "in the now"—without looking back or ahead—also took precedence.

Returning to the Scene — Flashbacks of Terror

A touch of post-traumatic stress shoots through my psyche and body in the form of increased anxiety each time I return to see my breast surgeon or other medical professionals.

The concern in others' eyes puts me in a heightened sense of alert. Once you've had a cancer diagnosis, I have observed that medical providers typically give more scrutiny to your health as a patient.

For example, extra menstrual bleeding was not considered "just the onset of menopause." I was offered drugs to stop it. Instead, I called my gynecologist who wisely listened thoroughly and explored possibilities that led to my being sent back to the hospital for a Dilation and Curettage (D&C) procedure to remove tissue from inside the uterus to stop the bleeding, my third surgery in six months. (Four months earlier I had a skin cancer removed, and two months before that procedure, my lumpectomy was performed.)

Fortunately, the D&C was routine with no additional abnormalities. Had I simply taken the drugs, I could have increased my risks for ovarian cancer, I later learned.

Staying centered in expectations for great health is a continual challenge when many healthcare providers—to cover all bases— are too quick to prescribe fear-based solutions based on old paradigms. As a patient committed to advocating for my own healthcare, I have often found it challenging to stay calm within the sterile environments of hospitals or doctor offices.

Additionally, health is just never taken for granted again. Once given a cancer diagnosis, you learn that life is unpredictable, that curveballs can come from anywhere.

Even though I had changed my diet and lifestyle to remain cancer-free, the anxiety of the first MRI seven months post-surgery caught me off-guard. I thought I would breeze through this testing. Instead, I found myself in the waiting room crying, flashing back to the previous year's test results, when I had been unsure if the intruder would be a death or life sentence.

To complete the patient data all over again spiraled me back to the day when I was first diagnosed. Surely, healthcare providers could find a way to avoid having patients duplicate this information each visit.

Luckily, my dear friend who drove me to the testing was a therapist. She ended up massaging my shoulders and doing other exercises to shift the energy and relax me while I waited to be called for the MRI.

On the very same day, my breast surgeon was kind enough to follow up, with the good news that everything on my MRI was clear. Celebrating that evening, I knew more deeply than ever, that good health is a gift. To continue enjoying it, I needed to monitor my thoughts, beliefs, stress levels, and environments—and spend as much time as possible in nurturing settings. Instead of recalling scary memories, I now needed to focus on creating new possibilities.

PART TWO:

EMBRACING A NEW MINDSET FOR LIVING

"Healing yourself, whether from heartbreak, illness, addiction, family struggles, or professional disappointment, is not for the faint of heart. It takes serious courage—Olympic courage—to do what it takes to transform pain into gold. I believe healing is possible, no matter what others say."

—Lissa Rankin, M.D., author of *Mind Over Medicine,* from her *Daily Flame* newsletter

STEPPING OFF THE CONVEYOR BELT...

From panic to power: the biggest decision of my life

I had to go deeper than I ever thought capable, and initiate a big pause in my life, to see if what these medical professionals advised resonated with my inner wisdom. With authority, and to help lessen the anxiety in choosing next steps, my medical team gave me up to a month to make a decision. Yet, no alternative approaches beyond radiation for healing were offered.

Giving myself permission to pause versus panic, I set the following guidelines for myself by disconnecting from all but the basic requirements of day-to-day living:

- **No more rambling "woe is me" conversations.**
- **No more dissecting the overload of technical medical information.**
- **No more focusing on scary "what if" mortality thoughts running through my mind.**

Instead, I would embrace long stretches of quiet, and patiently wait for answers to come forth from the guidance of my soul and Higher Power.

BECOMING YOUR AUTHORITY

"The intuitive mind is a sacred gift, and the rational mind is a faithful servant." –Physicist Albert Einstein

Surviving cancer, like many midlife challenges, can be a terribly lonely journey, even with the best support systems. If we instead see the disease as our soul's calling for growth, we can become our own authority, finally learning to take care of our bodies and create optimal health.

Much of conventional medicine is still based on old paradigms, but holistic approaches are not typically covered by health insurance or taken seriously by some in the medical profession.

No one can tell us with full assurance what is best for us—not even family members or friends who love us. We must take responsibility for what is best for our own bodies. We benefit our healing by taking the time to listen deep within for guidance. Day by day we must consistently balance medical opinions from trusted sources while also adhering to the innate healing wisdom of our bodies.

In the end, I made a tough, gut-wrenching choice that veered from some recommendations of the conventional path, declining the "gold plan" option of radiation and drug therapy with Tamoxifen that supposedly helps prevent recurrence. Instead, I opted to have the lump removed and heal myself with a healthy diet, lifestyle changes, and by using "energy as medicine," an approach even famous TV personality Dr. Mehmet Oz, cardiothoracic surgeon and Columbia University professor, employs and has touted as the wave of the future in healing.

For me, it was both an intelligent choice—based on asking tough questions—and a spiritual decision, sensing there was a much higher purpose where I would be sharing my experience of living from a new paradigm for health.

Whether using conventional medicine or not, these alternate healing routes will benefit even those who have never received a cancer diagnosis.

THE BIG PAUSE

I came to my choice by setting time alone to research. Suzanne Somers' book, *"Knockout,"* provided an excellent overview of alternative treatments from some leading-edge doctors who are curing cancer. I also recommend the book, *"Anti Cancer: A New Way of Life,"* by David Servan-Schreiber, M.D., Ph.D., who moved himself through a 15-year battle from brain cancer back to health.

During this time I asked questions of my doctors, learning that I could later opt for the conventional approach if a recurrence happened.

After all the research and talking with breast cancer survivors, I intentionally avoided contact with others for a few days while I allowed the right answer for me to come forth. Hours were spent walking the beach, with my eyes focused on the beauty around me. Nature is one of the best sanctuaries for accessing our innate wisdom and healing abilities. I accepted no phone calls and made no plans with friends. I wanted time alone to make this life-directing decision.

The heaviness of choosing to mix conventional and alternative care—and decide where one should leave off and another take over—was daunting. I later explained to friends:

> *"This isn't like deciding whether I should date a certain guy or not, or take on a specific project or job. This could be a life or death choice."*

I had two teenage children who I wanted to mother and also be a friend to in later life, and a grandmother to their children one day.

Sitting on the beach after my soul search, I re-opened Somers' book. On page 152, Dr. Russell Blaylock advised, when asked what a woman is to do if through an MRI or thermogram cancer is found:

> "If it were me, I would say I'm not having chemotherapy, and I'm not having radiation. I would let them surgically remove the tumor with a simple lumpectomy and then I would take care of the rest nutritionally."

Many other doctors I researched, along with two nutritionists who are also chiropractors, recommended the same.

Closing Somers' book, I felt the decision I had made hours earlier, independently of Dr. Blaylock's advice, was validated. I returned home clear in my choice, and kept my decision private and close to my heart for a while. I knew that no matter what happened, I was going to love myself and not judge myself wrong in any way for following my inner guidance.

This grueling inward journey, where I had to fight the continual urge to make a quick decision, felt akin to what I went through 11 years earlier in divorce. At that time, I spent many mornings walking the country road by our home crying, asking God for direction. The answer came in a short inner whisper while showering. *"You have suffered enough,"* were the words I heard. The answer to decline radiation also came in a soft whisper of *"Do nothing now,"* with a great peace that followed.

I cannot guarantee my choice will prevent the recurrence of breast cancer. Yet, neither can the doctors guarantee that the conventional "gold plan" of medical treatment (as the radiation/Tamoxifen treatment is referred to), can prevent a recurrence.

The "gold plan" can minimize a recurrence, but the long-lasting effects of radiation are still unclear. Tamoxifen can cause other kinds of cancer, not to mention weight gain and blood clots, I was told by others in healthcare.

Holding my soul-searching decision privately for a bit, I happened upon others who used conventional medicine. Some fared well; others did not. I spoke with one woman who went the traditional route, only to find out later the radiation may have hurt other parts of her body. Despite being told she would likely be cancer-free for "the next 40 years," she developed lung cancer, then a brain tumor, and died within a few years.

Yet, another woman—a nurse, treated with radiation and chemotherapy who had a double mastectomy—told me she is happily 14 years cancer-free. She, like many others, said her breast cancer had turned out to be a great gift. It taught her to slow down, and reorganize her life priorities.

My choice to decline radiation was not well received in the conventional medical community. My oncologist, who I later fired, suggested I was setting myself up for a worst-case scenario of later having metastatic breast cancer that could lead to death. My breast surgeon accepted the decision with caution, ordering additional mammograms and MRIs over the next year that came through clear.

Bucking external authority is not easy, especially for women who have been conditioned from early life to nurture, "be nice," and please others.

In fact, saying "no" is often a major step needed to increase self-esteem. In the raw vulnerability of a cancer diagnosis, it can be even more challenging to assert one's more powerful self. There are more of "them" in the room—the healthcare workers—than us the patient, who sometimes spend long periods of time alone in a johnny on an examination table waiting. We are also often looking up at our medical team as they check us out, exacerbating the feelings of powerlessness.

In so many ways, it is easier initially to "hand over" decisions to those trained in conventional medicine. Yet, the more I researched, the more I saw what those medical professionals could not teach me (because they are not trained to do so). You cannot just treat the symptoms; you need to treat the causes that brought about the disease. An emotional detox process is often needed to clear the stressors that led to the diagnosis in the first place.

In the end, for me, the choice to decline radiation became one of the most courageous and self-esteem building decisions of my life.

"Developing self-esteem requires an act of revolution, or several mini-revolutions, in which we begin to separate from group thought and establish our own sense of authority. We may suddenly realize we hold an opinion different from our family or our peers, but in either case we will have difficulty freeing ourselves from the group's energy, whose strength depends upon numbers and opposition to most expressions of individuality. The act of finding our own voice, even in mini-revolutions, is spiritually significant."

—Caroline Myss, medical intuitive, best-selling author, and internationally renowned speaker.

BECOMING PROACTIVE

What's Next?

What does one do to prevent recurrence when they have declined radiation?

I took it on, almost as a second full-time job, to learn of every healing approach I could to help my body reach optimal health again. Studies show survivors do best when they take full responsibility for their own health, not just deferring to doctors to "make them well."

By veering off the conventional path, continuing to act on strong intuition and extensive research, I discovered several complementary healing approaches that calm the body and elevate the mind to greater states of love. Even for those who accept traditional and conventional medical routes, these holistic approaches can assist in increasing longevity.

Love is the highest state of energy, from which miraculous healings are possible, according to Dr. David Hawkins, M.D., Ph.D., author of *Letting Go: The Pathway of Surrender.* To reach that state as frequently as I could, I used tools and techniques from the emerging fields of epigenetics and neuroscience, training with some of the best, including Dr. Joe Dispenza and Deepak Chopra, through his powerful meditation series on "perfect health."

I also learned ways to release the emotional toxins and unhealthy beliefs that contribute to illness, and block continued healing. Finding groups of like-minded others committed to taking charge of their health, and connecting to the power of the collective unconscious, accelerated my healing journey.

I now share these "hidden jewels" of groups and healing centers across the country, where one can stop in and receive, for no charge, amazing healing opportunities.

No matter what route you choose, shedding past emotional stressors and living from a place of love and worthiness, is paramount to creating your positive outcome.

THE BEGINNINGS OF USING "ENERGY AS MEDICINE"

"We're beginning now to understand things that we know in our hearts were true but could not measure. As we get better at understanding how little we know about the body, we begin to realize that the next big frontier in medicine is energy medicine. It's not the mechanistic parts of the joints moving. It's not the chemistry of our bodies. It's understanding, for the first time, how energy influences how we feel."

—Dr. Mehmet Oz, November 20, 2007, The Oprah Show

Walk gently with me, dear reader, and bring an open mind, as I describe my unique healing experience using "energy as medicine."

When we align with others who have similar intentions for good health, we can tap into what is referred to as "the collective unconscious," a power far greater than our individual ego selves. This expanded state of being can also complement and/or exceed the limits of conventional medicine and pharmaceutical-based approaches to healing, as evidenced in numerous studies shared later in this book.

1. TONG REN® Healing Circles: Hope, Love and Miracle Healings ...Opening the Mind to the Power of the Collective Unconscious

With much trepidation—and still in a high state of anxiety post-cancer diagnosis and surgery—I entered my first Tong Ren healing circle at the suggestion of a wise and loving friend. In the past, I had declined such invitations, thinking this "Chinese quackery" was not for me. Yet, my cancer scare opened me to new ways of thinking. With a renewed commitment to life, I became willing to explore new options to bring my body back in balance at a cellular level.

Created by a prominent Boston healer and acupuncturist, Tom Tam, these Tong Ren healing circles commenced in 2001 for treating cancer in Quincy, Massachusetts, and have been attended by thousands searching for relief from a variety of illnesses and ailments. Many have been successfully healed, or able to return to living a normal life.

Sitting on a folding chair in a circle of about 20 people in a garage-like setting of a fitness firm in Topsfield, Massachusetts, I watched practitioners and participants tap with a hammer on a plastic doll, on areas that would be Chinese meridian points in a human, to release blockages in the body.

What the hell am I doing here? I thought to myself. *I will never tell anyone what I'm doing every Tuesday night.*

This reaction surprised me, for I have used Emotional Freedom Technique (EFT)—another healing tool that taps on Chinese meridian points—in my coaching practice. Watching a doll be tapped however, as each person in the circle told of their ailments or discomforts, simply felt weird.

Slowly I began observing the color in some faces change to a healthier red, while I heard others say they felt the energy surge as increased warmth in their bodies. Tom Tam described this energy as "Qi" (also spelled Chi), the life force of the collective unconscious from others in the room and beyond, moving throughout the body. With an intention for healing—and an openness to receiving the Qi accelerated by this healing approach—the energy heightens. Or, put another way, the removal of the blockage through tapping on the doll's meridian point helps restore the nature flow of energy so the body can correct itself and heal.

Likened to "acupuncture without the needles," Tong Ren healing directs energy from the collective or transpersonal mind to relieve physical, emotional, or spiritual conditions.

Bravely, each person in the room continued to disclose their ailments, allowing others to tap on the doll directly where that ailment is represented. Tom Tam believes it is these blockages—the unbalanced bioelectricity of the body—that cause illness, as opposed to the strictly chemical causes cited by conventional Western medicine.

"Western medicine focuses on the biochemistry [versus bioelectricity] of the body, where money can be made by using chemicals versus employing natural healing techniques," Tam claims.

Lifestyle changes and movement also can be effective in accelerating healing, because "cancer cannot thrive in well-oxygenated cells," he says. Yoga, Tai Chi, Chi Gong, Reiki, massage, and acupuncture are a few methods he suggests, adding, "The phrenic nerve on the neck is responsible for oxygen, and you want to keep the neck free." He attributes rising cancer rates to our lifestyles. "Today, there is more tension in the upper back and the neck. Computers and cell phones add to cancer rates rising, not because of radiation as people think, but because of our posture. The way we sit in front of a computer strains our neck and back, as does the way we hold a cell phone."

Initially, I was fearful in attending a Tong Ren session that hearing others' health problems would leave me depressed. Instead I began seeing all of us in the room as one, with an incredible indomitable spirit to live. The love and compassion in the circle far exceeded what I had felt in the outside world. I witnessed genuine love in the form of the tenderness of husbands and wives sitting side-by-side in support of one another, the newly diagnosed embraced by kindness, and then applause after hearing a Stage-IV tumor had lessened or disappeared.

When it came my turn to disclose my illness, I shared that I recently had a lumpectomy on my right breast. I then let them know I was choosing to decline radiation and Tamoxifen, opting instead to make diet and lifestyle changes—as a researched recommendation for early-stage breast cancer.

"Good for you," a participant remarked. "Stay strong. You're doing the right thing." His comment amazed me, for it was the first time anyone validated my internal *knowing* that for now I needed to honor my tumor-free body.

Still, during that first night and the subsequent one, I did not feel any significant change. Slowly, I found each time I went, I slept soundly for the first time since hearing my diagnosis. My face and neck would grow warm, and I began to feel the Qi energy. Suppressed emotions came forth and I found myself later privately gushing tears of release.

This release is important to letting go of blockages in the body. The subsequent Tui Na massages I did solo with a Tong Ren practitioner also helped me further release emotions and blockages.

For three years, I attended Tong Ren healing circles once or twice a week. At times it felt a nuisance, as I would have preferred to be wining and dining with friends. Yet, the alternative of radiation and putting unnecessary drugs into my body felt like a worse option.

Plus, as much as I love and am enormously grateful for my dear friends, the post-cancer journey benefits from a connection with those who have been through similar healing challenges.

Tom Tam's Tong Ren circles were my initial safe place to honor my belief in my body's innate ability to heal with proper care, nutrition, and the power of the collective unconscious. It kept me committed to living in renewed and more vibrant health.

To find a Tong Ren class in your area, visit:
www.tomtam.com/guinea-pig-class-directory/

2. THE MIND BODY PROGRAM FOR CANCER, Benson-Henry Institute for Mind Body Medicine at Massachusetts General Hospital, Boston

Reducing stress and enhancing resiliency

The first three months after a cancer diagnosis represent the most critical juncture of the healing journey. According to a study by S. Greer, referenced in the workbook from The Mind Body Program for Cancer at Massachusetts General Hospital's renowned Benson-Henry Institute:

> "Of major importance was the finding that at the 5-,10-, and 15-year follow-ups, the best single predictor of death (from any cause, including breast cancer) or recurrence of cancer was the psychological response of each woman three months after surgery. Her mental attitude three months after surgery better predicted the likelihood of dying or having a recurrence of breast cancer than did the size of her tumor, the tumor's histologic grade, or her age. Women who show fighting spirit ('I'm going to beat this') or denial ('I never had cancer, the doctor took my breast as a precaution') had a 50 percent chance of surviving 15 years in good health. Women with the other three attitudes (stoic acceptance, hopelessness, anxious preoccupation) had about a 15 percent chance of surviving 15 years."

A few weeks into attending the Tong Ren healing circles, a participant mentioned, "Tong Ren helps a lot, but The Mind Body Program at Massachusetts General Hospital changed my life. I had been under so much stress, divorce, bankruptcy, you name it."

I, too, had been under severe stress for three years prior to my cancer diagnosis, and despite what conventional medical doctors told me, I believe it played a significant role in my getting ill. I also believe early childhood trauma affected my health at a cellular level—or at least the way I conditioned myself to respond to challenges after living in fight-or-flight mode, psychologically "running" from a schizophrenic mother.

Looking at this kind Tong Ren participant, I was intrigued, for this now cancer-free man, had been given a death sentence nine years prior for Stage-IV throat cancer. I handed him my business card, and the next day received contact information for Dr. Ann Webster, director of The Mind/Body Program at Massachusetts General Hospital at the time.

As part of the screening process, I learned the program was not a therapy group, but rather a place for learning techniques and skills to deal with stress through and beyond cancer. Listening carefully to my inner knowing, and bypassing all my resistance, I chose to make healing myself my number one priority. Great time and financial sacrifice was involved, yet in the long-term, investing in my health was the best gift I could give my children and myself. Plus, like many women (and cancer survivors), I finally had to learn to put myself first.

8 Characteristics of Long-Term Cancer Survivors

1. They are realistic and accept their diagnosis but do not take it as a death sentence.
2. They have a fighting spirit and refuse to be helpless/hopeless.
3. They have changed lifestyles.
4. They are assertive and have the ability to get out of stressful and unproductive situations.
5. They are tuned in to their own psychological and physical needs, and they take care of them.
6. They are able to talk openly about their illness.
7. They have a sense of personal responsibility for their health, and they look at treating the physician as a collaborator.
8. They are altruistically involved with other persons with cancer.

As given in a handout to participants of The Mind Body Program for Cancer.

My writing business and coaching practice gave me the flexibility to handle the weekly trips to Boston, which with travel time, entailed a half-day commitment each Monday for ten weeks. Continually I had to trust there would be payback for these efforts, reminding myself that I was worth this investment. Dealing with career and money issues could temporarily be delayed. Postponing attending to my health could not wait.

Entering the roomful of other cancer survivors at the renowned Benson-Henry Institute for Mind Body Medicine of Massachusetts General Hospital in October 2012, I felt both relief and trepidation.

Finally, I had found a safe place to regroup from the past five months of rushing around with adrenaline to live every moment to the fullest, or what I dubbed my "hurry up and slow down" phase. I knew I needed to rest, but I did not want to miss a minute of life.

At the same time, I was not fully ready to admit that I had cancer, for in my mind, I was creating a healthy new body. Being with others who had cancer made my past health challenge real. I did not want to call any extra attention to the earlier diagnosis, but neither did I want to deny what I had just been through. Honoring all parts of the journey was crucial to my well-being.

My friends were, and continued to be, incredibly loving and supportive. Yet, I also needed to share with others who had gone through a similar ordeal, to help further awaken me from a death scare. Besides, almost universally, most cancer survivors have stories of those who flee from our lives or ignore our changed state upon hearing of our cancer diagnoses. Looking back, I, too, had been guilty of not engaging as fully as I could have with health-challenged friends, fearing that talking of their disease would be too depressing or scary.

For me, accepting that I once had cancer, changed my psyche, confronted my will to live, and clarified my life purpose. Instead of feeling abandoned by those who could not comprehend the new types of support I needed, I created a sense of belonging by seeking out like-minded others who were uplifting and inspiring.

While there were many light-hearted moments during the 10-week program, I also felt a seriousness and professionalism behind the facilitation and workbook that helped validate the intensity of what I had just gone through.

Thanks to the coaching expertise and new skills and techniques taught by Dr. Webster, my hugest gain was learning to be still for 20 minutes a day and feel all the emotions I had repressed. As participants, we were required to meditate daily and keep journal sheets of our progress. Our stress levels were also tested at the beginning and end of program, and significantly shifted for many of us.

"Self-care and being with other people going through the same thing is extremely important," said Dr. Webster, who believes strongly that face-to-face contact is very healing. "People are too isolated today," she observes.

MGH TIPS

1. Change your behavior and eliminate worry by focusing on the present moment while in conversation, walking, eating, listening, or bathing/showering. Appreciate that "being" is healthier than "doing."

2. Get out of isolation and build rich friendships. Women without close friends are four times as likely to die from the disease than women with 10 or more friends.

3. Embrace the unknown. Your psyche has been changed forever once you get a diagnosis. To create a new mindset for living, give yourself permission to stay for long periods in the unknown.

Five elements of the training include instruction in relaxation, yoga, cognitive therapy, mindfulness, and resiliency.

"The most important component is for the patients to learn to elicit the relaxation response of quiet," Dr. Webster says. "It's the foundation of everything to learn to quiet the body and mind before we can make any kind of change. Stress and anxiety is not good for the immune system. Decreasing stress gives the immune system a boost."

The cognitive therapy techniques, based on years of research, help patients shift their thoughts and beliefs. "Cognitive therapy enables people to see they are creating their own problems with their thinking and once they see that, it's illuminating," she says, carefully adding, "There are certain negative thoughts though that are 100 percent okay, and that we just need to accept. For example, it's justifiable to be upset about having cancer, but you don't have to stay stuck on the thought 24 hours a day. You want to focus on living, being, and finding some optimism."

The results from the mind-body techniques have been so profound that Dr. Webster created her own documentary, "Everything Matters," which includes interviews with five patients, all of whom were told they did not have long to live. They are all alive now, 5, to 15 and 28-plus years later.

Resiliency is also an important part of the program, because some participants had other "horrible things" besides cancer happen to them. One gentleman's wife left him two weeks after his cancer diagnosis. Another woman with two adopted children had cancer three times, and her husband left her. The skills of resiliency allowed these participants to cope and move beyond the negative aspects of their situations, and recover optimum health.

After decades of living and preaching self-care, Dr. Webster offers this advice for cancer survivors:

1. Examine every single thing you can do to maintain your health. You have to change everything in your mind and body.
2. Eat well—get chemicals and hormones out of your food.
3. Create social supports around you.
4. Rest.
5. Get calm.
6. Slow down. "Everyone is stressed beyond belief. Everybody needs to slow down."

7. Do the things that are most important to you.
8. If you are unhappy in a job or relationship, get out of it.

As a participant of Dr. Webster's program in 2012, I can attest that it is indeed a gentle environment in which to direct the body to heal in new ways. Dr. Webster led our group with grace, compassion, non-judgment, and as an exemplary model of calm.

Stepping into More Power
...insights from other participants interviewed

(In this section, names of participants have been changed to protect their privacy. Sadly, many shared with me that they feared ever getting hired again if a potential employer knew of their cancer diagnosis. One was told companies do not want to absorb the insurance risk. Although illegal to discriminate, it is hard to know the real reason sometimes for not getting hired).

Patient #1 – A Woman of Action Empowers Herself

At the last meeting of our Mind Body Program for Cancer in January 2013, Mona, a 55-year-old global communications executive and former Boston broadcast journalist, handed us each a dark chocolate candy bar with a bow on top. "Life is a gift," she said as we received our treat.

A year earlier, Mona had been diagnosed with Chronic Lymphocytic Leukemia, otherwise known as CLL. She was told at the time that there is no known cure (although through alternative health care approaches she was able to keep her white blood counts down and renew her energy (*see related Chapter on Tong Ren Healing*).

"The doctor told me the diagnosis immediately and matter-of-factly after waiting six to seven weeks to get test results," she said. "I kept asking questions to get information, like what do I need to do? No one had any answers. No website. Nothing. I was only left with an appointment for an MRI and a follow-up in four months and told to wear a mask in public if I was out with a lot of people, like on an airplane."

Determined, she researched online resources for help, and came up with a loss until through "word-of-mouth serendipity" a friend told her of The Mind Body Program for Cancer at MGH. Not ever seeing herself as a helpless person, she empowered herself to join the group.

Trust your gut.

"When I first went to the program, we didn't know much about each other, but I saw faces of people I knew I had something in common with," she shared. "The jury was out if I was in the right place at the right time, but a little voice inside my head said, 'You're exactly where you need to be in this moment.' Dr. Webster was excellent at assuring that this was not a 'woe is me' class."

Still, she was admittedly scared when she heard of others' diagnoses and medical conditions.

However, at the second session her feelings shifted. "I learned it was not about bemoaning what was wrong with us, but about embracing life and how we can live it better," she explained.

Then she was thrown another curveball, just before the third class, when she was told she had a fast-progressing form of CLL. "I was at the class, but not really present," Mona says. "Being in shock was unusual for me, given I am a crisis expert who can handle everything."

Returning to the program kept her grounded so after the fourth class, she realized she was now looking forward to attending each week.

"People understood one another's challenges even though they were not discussed," she says. "You need to have hope and know you are not alone and the only one out there."

Instead of hearing fearful stories, Mona witnessed participants' attitudes changing to the point where the group was suddenly "cheering and caring" for one another.

Build a team of positive people.

"I was able to be my normal self, and learned to monitor reactions later like when they found leukemia in my colon," she shared. Staying positive continues be a big part of Mona's life as she distances from negative people who drain her energy.

She also learned to live in the now and change her words when she responds to health inquiries. Instead of "Great, considering..." or "what if," she answers, "I feel great," if she does feel that in the moment.

Acting spontaneously also helps her seize the moment. During the blizzard of 2013, instead of nestling at home, she opted to venture out to the Four Seasons Hotel (she lives near it in Boston) to meet her girlfriend and the new beau who was trying to impress her. "I decided to throw caution to the wind and go meet them for drinks," she said. "I didn't like the bill later, but what the heck."

Mona's priorities also shifted. A former workaholic, she didn't even know she had any symptoms because fatigue felt so normal. Functioning on two to four hours of sleep a night, eating a handful of trail mix for dinner on the run, and living on airplanes had been her life before.

"I loved my career, but self-love and love for my family, for husband, come first now," Mona said. "I am still here, which is much more important than my career and job I was losing health over."

She was particularly impressed by the way the program shifted her way of being. "This class was a wonderful part of my journey forward emotionally, developmentally, and in making progress toward helping myself," Mona claimed. "It is not only the medical profession that helps me, but we all have to help ourselves with our own care. The Mind Body Program was an opening to learn how I could find the resources and ways on my path to do my part in my recovery."

Patient #2 – A strong woman of great faith, inspiring others with gratitude

"I'm not contagious."—Pat says in sharing her cancer diagnosis with her grandchild.

Pat's kindness and grace belie the many challenges she has endured. Like many cancer survivors I have come to know, she had a lot of trauma in her life prior to her diagnosis of Stage-IV lymphoma in her leg in 2009.

Three years before her diagnosis, her house caught on fire following a flood and had to be gutted. *(That time period is significant, as both a well-known cancer therapist and my second opinion surgeon have observed, many women experience a time of incredible stress three years prior to being diagnosed with breast cancer.)*

Pat also shared another common characteristic of some cancer survivors—she worked in the "helping professions" as a nurse in community and public health her entire adult life. Many in the helping professions overextend themselves in caring for others at the expense of themselves and their own health. Learning to be kind and nurturing to themselves first can be part of the healing. Eventually, Pat could only work part-time due to chronic fatigue and immune system deficiencies that forced her to spend entire summers in bed resting. She is now 72.

Her trials continued. Pat lost one brother who was found dead in the bathtub due to a heart attack, just a month before her diagnosis and another brother to a heart attack, a month after she was diagnosed.

Her earlier life was also challenging, losing a schizophrenic brother to suicide after he jumped off the Golden Gate Bridge when Pat was 30. She grew up with an alcoholic father and was the oldest of five children. Her mother later died of breast cancer and her father of Alzheimer's disease after a long life, leaving her alone with her sister.

"I was always in fight-or-flight, which affects the adrenal glands," Pat explains. "It's like a valve stays open. I am still not totally unwound, with all the work I've done. I still feel myself stressing."

The Mind Body Program for Cancer was one of the doors she believed God opened for her after getting diagnosed with lymphoma. The chemotherapy and radiation treatments were far worse than the diagnosis itself, she says, due to the many side effects including: neurological episodes which she thought were strokes, high blood pressure, and experiencing periods of not being able to talk.

"The Mind Body Program for Cancer was wonderful," Pat said. "I'm doing relaxation exercises pretty regularly now. I liked the mini stress-reducing techniques we were taught, the daily 'feel goods' and the program got me back into journaling again."

Pat especially enjoyed learning to be present to the moment, seeing the benefits of slowing down. "The program helped me focus on the mind-body connection of the now. We live in such a hurried world and it is important to have excellence... and excellence sometimes takes time," she says. "We're meant to be gracious and do things with joy and purpose, enjoy the now, the beauty of nature, the little animals and little children."

She also attributes increased feelings of self-love as part of her own healing journey.

During her initial stages of treating cancer, she asked many who deal with moment-to-moment: "What is my source of being preyed upon with cancer?" **She was told three thought patterns contributed to her illness** (which my own energy healers also validated later in this book):

1. **Self-hatred**
2. **Unworthiness**
3. **A death wish**

She prayed to heal any subconscious beliefs around these thoughts and continued to practice self-love through meditating, yoga, and one-on-one healing sessions with Dr. Ann Webster, director of the Program.

Connection to others going through a similar healing journey was a key benefit of the Program, although at first Pat (like the other program participants shared) was resistant to talking about it. "There is so much strength in unified, community love, which I've seen again and again on a personal level," she states.

She also now lives with a heightened awareness of goodness and gratitude. "Cancer made me more aware of everything," she noted.

Patient #3 – A woman of hope and compassion

The Mind Body Program for Cancer taught Nadia, a breast cancer survivor in her 50s, to be even more compassionate with herself.

"It helped me understand the stress I had been carrying, and gave me tools to use over time to adjust to it and bring the stress down more quickly," Nadia explained. "And I never felt anything but support. Everybody in their own way chimed in."

The program was especially helpful after her chemotherapy treatments ended, and all the love and support she felt from her hospital medical team checking in on her daily was suddenly gone.

> *"It's like when you take a class, and you finish all your papers and take the final exam," she said, adding, "You feel lost afterward."*

Her support group at the hospital was loving and helpful, particularly around sharing "tribal knowledge" of treatments, she said. Yet, The Mind Body Program for Cancer differed by teaching skills for reducing stress versus focusing on symptoms.

Nadia said she thrived from the caring nature of Dr. Webster, who took the time to write encouraging notes on the class member's weekly journal sheets, and the safe, non-judgmental environment she creates.

"Definitely do the group. Many don't understand that it will help them release stress, tension, and worry," Nadia urged. "You need to be able to talk in a setting where people understand, unlike family, who unless they've been through it, cannot understand. They have their own agenda, schedules, kids to take care of. It's like going to grad school or war or going through it together. You can be yourself."

> *"Others inaccurately perceive that having a cancer diagnosis means you're going to die soon, when in fact, many survive longer than ever before due to advances in treatments and testing."*

During her treatments she felt loved and "carried" by all those friends and medical personnel who cared for her. "It was total trust, and they were all walking by my side," she says. "With chemo you have to let down and let your whole body take over and you can't do anything else."

She also relied on the patience of self-love and faith that God has everything under control. "Self-love means taking care of yourself," she states. "There's a reason this happened. I love myself despite the bad thing I'm going through."

Regardless of how challenging her treatment days were, she always wanted to offer encouragement to others—especially those who lost their hair, who she says have the most difficult time. "I didn't care how bad I felt on a day of chemo. Even when I couldn't stand five minutes without feeling like I'd faint, I'd focus on sending courage to them."

Today, she wants to continue extending her passion for helping people by creating a new career supporting cancer patients.

Like the other Mind Body Program patients interviewed, Nadia no longer has tolerance for negative people. "I have been given a gift of life so I don't want to spend time with negative people."

Other changes she has observed about herself include:

- less patience for nonsense
- less tolerance for inequities such as someone living in a $40 million home who does not "give back"
- not trying to solve the world's problems
- speaking up more

"I am flexible and adaptable, but I won't work nights anymore," she said of her new priority of a more balanced life. "A lot of people are out of control in their lives and are willing to do anything to the detriment of their own health."

3. DR. JOE DISPSENZA - Neuroscience as a healing tool

"The latest research supports the notion that we have a natural ability to change the brain and body by thought alone, so that it looks biologically the same, like some future event has already happened. Because you can make thought real more than anything else, you can change who you are from brain cell to gene, given the right understanding." —Dr. Joe Dispenza

Two lonely years into this courageous, scary journey as a pioneer for my own health, I came across a book that changed my life: *You Are the Placebo: Making Your Mind Matter,* by Dr. Joe Dispenza. Up until that point, I had been acting solely on intuition, without any clear direction for healing beyond the dismal recommendations from the conventional medical community and an occasional visit to a naturopathic doctor.

Many times, I felt it would have been much easier to do the recommended radiation treatments and take the suggested Tamoxifen drug than to accept responsibility for designing my own healing path. Yet that soft and ever-expanding, wise voice inside kept saying, *"No, not now."*

Fortunately, Dr. Dispenza's work gave me a meditation practice I could follow to keep my mind aligned with my body's innate ability to heal. More importantly, it validated my inner knowing. Suddenly, I felt I had a companion on this journey.

A successful chiropractor and lecturer, Dr. Dispenza lives what he teaches. He trained his own mind to heal his body after getting run over by a SUV in 1986 while participating in a Palm Springs triathlon. He later followed through on a commitment to himself to study neuroscience, and is now considered a renowned expert on change, the brain, and human potential.

Using his work, many followers have achieved miraculous healing, while others have manifested financial abundance and fulfilled dreams.

"Stay open to the unexpected, and be prepared for surprises as the mind recalibrates to new possibilities. Begin by being grateful now for the event you want to happen," he urges.

Initially, I committed 45 days to listening to his 55-minute CD that accompanied the book. At first, I would stir restlessly, not wanting to sit still that long to complete a daily session. Increasingly, I became more patient and felt calmer, but nothing outwardly significantly changed—or so I thought.

Then, one morning two months after beginning the meditations, I literally bumped into a man while walking on a curvy part of a road near the ocean path. We agreed to meet for lunch, and then dated a bit before he moved across the country to Arizona. Several months later, at his invitation, I joined him there, 3,000 miles away from everything I had ever known.

I could never have scripted this chapter of my new life story. I believe living in a state of expanded consciousness through my daily meditations opened my mind to new possibilities and elevated levels of courage.

Arizona was my new start of reinventing myself post-cancer, and aligning with like-minded others committed to spirituality and health in the ways I am. I had to leave behind everything that was familiar, and place myself in a new environment to live from the new consciousness I had so diligently integrated through the meditations. I later had to do even more shedding of old ways to find my true essence.

New England, with all its beauty and familiar friends and family, will always hold a special place in my heart. Yet, no matter how hard I tried to shift my circumstances and inner being, I felt stuck in old stories of stress and survival.

Environments matter

I am not the same person I was in New England. In moving to Scottsdale, Arizona, I made a choice to live from peace. My lakeside condo, where I did most of my reinventing, gave me a tranquility to rediscover who I was without the childhood conditioning that previously defined me.

Little did I know, but that move allowed me to attend a "Progressive Weekend" in person with Dr. Joe Dispenza in Tempe, Arizona, integrating even more of his latest neuroscience research into my healing journey and coaching business.

The moment I arrived, I felt bliss, knowing a grace was surrounding me as I committed to exploring my essence in new ways. For the next two evenings and days, we meditated collectively. The focus was on shifting from the negative survivor emotions (such as guilt, fear, and worry), to the more empowering elevated emotions of creating (like joy, love, and gratitude).

The shifts and insights were incredible, particularly because Dr. Dispenza explained in great detail, with supporting evidence, the science behind the guided meditations set to music. That knowledge made the group experience even more powerful.

Some moments entailed tearful releases in the wee hours of the evening. One meditation ignited a "life in review" for me, contrasting the old life I was conditioned to live and the new one I was creating. At other times during the weekend, we practiced breath work at the beginning of meditation that was especially powerful, almost as if I could feel the emotional toxins of a lifetime of stress leave my body.

Embracing the unknown, and surrendering to a power greater than myself, became paramount to shifting into more vibrant states of being. I later dubbed this stage "a blind date with destiny," letting go of control and releasing all that was familiar opened up unlimited possibilities for a new life.

Each time we meditated, I was determined to claim my new life as a healthy, prosperous teacher and best-selling author, who lived from the beliefs that I AM ENOUGH and I AM WANTED. The latter belief of feeling WANTED was more significant to me than knowing I AM LOVED, having felt a lifetime of rejection as the daughter of a schizophrenic mom and the limiting subconscious-driven choices I made as a result.

Through ongoing healing and continual trusting of my innate wisdom, I came to know that cancer is *not* my story. Living life in a new way, from a love-based consciousness is the calling I am here to deliver. The frightened young girl could stop running and rest now. A self-empowered woman has taken over.

4. THE LITTLE CHAPEL, Paradise Valley, Arizona

Spontaneously healed into a new life mission

"God did not create us to suffer. He created us to be expressions of His love and light here on earth. Problems are great opportunities to grow if we look for the lessons they impart." —Sara Buckner O'Meara

Many who live in Arizona are not aware of The Little Chapel, a hidden jewel where people from all over the world and walks of life come to deepen their faith and experience miracle healings.

Two years after my divinely guided move to Arizona, a new friend asked me to join her in attending a Christmas healing service at The Little Chapel in Paradise Valley, led by Sara O'Meara.

Sara, with her friend, Yvonne Fedderson (who opens the services with announcements and prayer) has been offering healing services for more than 35 years. Yvonne hosts and provides a free fellowship luncheon that follows each service.

The two women met as actresses decades before on the set of *The Adventures of Ozzie and Harriet* and have been best friends ever since. For close to six decades they have been devoting their lives to helping victims of child abuse and neglect through leading the nonprofit organization they co-founded, Childhelp, which has programs and services throughout the country (www.childhelp.org). Both Sara and Yvonne have been nominated for The Nobel Peace Prize for rescuing more than 10 million children.

The Chapel is situated amidst beautiful gardens, and has a hand-painted angel mural along with other artistic touches that add a sense of serenity and beauty.

I thought mostly that I was attending a holiday event. I also brought another friend with me who was recovering from hip replacement surgery that same week.

Sara, I later learned, had a spontaneous healing from incurable cancer 40 years ago. Through that miracle, she believes she received unique and powerful guidance to help others.

At the end of the service, she called forth many to share their own testimonies or miracle healings that occurred while they were at services at this "Little Chapel." One pastor flew in from Hawaii to share his experience in being healed from cancer. Others got up and walked to the stage without pain for the first time in years from previous chronic issues.

I have gone to six other healing services of Sara's since and witnessed many others who spoke of being healed of back injuries, joint pains, "brokenness" (financially and otherwise), and lung issues. **About 80 percent of those who take part in the Little Chapel ministry are blessed with a profound healing miracle, according to Sara.**

Sara is quick to point out consistently that the credit for the healings belongs to God. She is only the conduit for bringing people together "of whatever faith, who seek peace, solace and communion with God." She spends hours preparing her service, and the day before she stays in full prayer, often getting inner guidance on who will appear at the service the following day and what suffering they may be enduring.

"In sharing my personal story and the tale of others who have been made whole through The Little Chapel ministry, I seek to shine a spotlight on the greatest physician, psychologist, and wellness practitioner the world has ever known: The Holy Spirit," Sara shares in her book, *Miracle Healing: God's Call.*

Sara's story

As a young woman with a family and her rewarding mission of advocating for children, her busy life took a sharp turn. She was diagnosed with an aggressive form of breast cancer that spread throughout her body, and she was given three months to live.

Lying in a hospital bed feeling hopeless and cheated by life, she heard a mesmerizing booming voice from the TV set, from Evangelist Kathryn Kuhlman, saying, "If you need a miracle come to Shrine Auditorium this Sunday." Growing up Presbyterian, Sara thought such healing services were "holy roller" affairs, theatrical and silly. Yet, the message stuck with her.

As she and many others who face mortality often decide, she opted to stay open-minded to all healing possibilities. She convinced her doctor to let her leave the hospital earlier than the four days he mandated, never telling him where she was going. She just had an operation with a 36" incision, which was clamped together to heal. She was told she could bleed to death if she moved.

Miraculously, on February 20, 1972, she got to the Shrine Auditorium in Los Angeles, California (as she lived nearby at the time). The auditorium was completely full, but a friend unexpectedly offered her a seat. With blood dripping from her body, she climbed to the vacant balcony chair. Suddenly, she was struck by a strange sense of lightness, like her body was lifted up and she hovered above looking down. She saw a pink cloud with the consistency of cotton candy in her peripheral vision.

Then, Kuhlman suddenly stopped her service and claimed, "There is a healing of a girl with cancer riddled throughout her body." The evangelist continued the service and stopped again, saying "This girl in the balcony is being healed. She is having a phenomenal experience. She feels a thousand needles going through her at the moment." She noted where Sara was sitting, and the color of her red dress. "God has saved you for a very special purpose. You are anointed," Kuhlman declared.

Concurrently, Sara felt as if needles were coursing through her skin, like an electric current. The entire row where she was sitting fell over like dominos in the seated position, feeling the overflow of the Holy Spirit going through her, she believes. She also thinks God's grace gave her a second chance at living.

X-rays confirmed Sara's cancer was gone. Similar to Dorothy's realization in the Wizard of Oz that the power was within all along, Sara became aware of her conduit abilities through Kuhlman during her healing and this began their subsequent mentorship. Sara later served Kuhlman by providing testimony at her events about the before and after healing experiences. Sara also began seeing light around the person who God would touch and heal during a service.

A year after Sara's healing, Kuhlman passed away. Then, a year after Kuhlman's death, a famous healing priest, Father Ralph DiOrio from Massachusetts, began doing research on Kuhlman and wanted to meet Sara. After meeting, he confirmed that God granted Sara with the gift of healing and that she must use it. Sara continued to hone her healing gift with Father DiOrio. On August 31, 1981, while at a team ministry with him, an image of a perfect white cross (which a photographer captured—and the photo is the book referenced at the end of this chapter) surrounded Sara.

The Little Chapel—Tidbits of information

The chair Sara was sitting in when the healing occurred was later purchased by her late husband, Colonel Robert Sigholtz, and is now placed on a small platform in the Little Chapel. The chapel is maintained through love, prayers, and voluntary donations and is incorporated as a non-profit entity.

At the Christmas healing service, Sara also gave each one of us in attendance a beautiful carved stone that said, "May there always be an angel beside you." It was wrapped in a gorgeous Christmas stocking.

Her first Little Chapel started in 1987 in Tarzana, California, with donations from friends who had been healed from Sara's ministry. She began it as her dream to offer a place of serenity dedicated to the glory of God, where people of all faiths could join together in worship and receive God's healing grace.

Sara's healing ministry continues to attract hundreds each month, with many standing outside or in an overflow room to experience the miracles that often occur within.

For me, attending the service helps keep me grounded in the connection of like-minded others who believe in the possibility of healing. I also use it to deepen my own faith in God. Belief is such a huge part of Sara's message each time. When someone experiences a healing, she asks if that person truly believes he or she has been healed.

For years, I also witnessed from leading healing and meditation circles that when we align with others committed to the same purpose or intention, results can be accelerated.

Adding faith, which can increase through the many testimonials heard at Sara's services, is another powerful component to wellness—especially for those newly diagnosed who, under stress and shock of hearing the scary "C" word, may have temporarily lost trust in their body's power to heal.

Asked how her spontaneous healing changed her life personally, Sara shared:

> "Getting a second chance at life made me want to give others a second chance as well. My faith was already deep but this experience took it to a new level, engaging my heart in a healing mission, acknowledging myself as a vessel through which God could work and committing my whole being to continuing my work with abused and neglected children.
>
> On the personal side of things, I believe those around you are naturally enriched when you are infused with a fresh

perspective on life and living totally in the light of God's grace. Mothering and all aspects of life are changed. You give with renewed love but you also know new boundaries and give love to yourself as well.

When we are awakened to God's miracles, we open our eyes like never before and all aspects of life come into focus. Your purpose ceases to be personal (self-serving) and evolves into a more divine spirit (serving God)."

Sara also offered these words of hope for those who are newly diagnosed with cancer:

"First of all, a diagnosis is never a death sentence. I have been told to settle my affairs and say goodbye to my family, but here I am all these decades later with so much more to accomplish. There is no doctor, nurse, family member, or friend who can tell when it's your time. Only God knows; He is the greatest physician. Fight this disease with a loving support system of medicine, education, but above all, God. Cancer is only a pausing point for the Holy Spirit to do some of His most important work in your life. Embrace the journey and believe in His plan for your health, healing and spiritual growth."

For more information about Sara's work,
or to attend a service, please email:
solittlechapel@gmail.com or call 480-922-4870.

The Little Chapel is located at 6135 E. Palo Verde Lane, Paradise Valley, AZ. The book that describes Sara's work, authored by Yvonne Fedderson, is *Miracle Healing: God's Call,* which shares more than 100 proven miracles that have taken place and been sustained at her Little Chapel. Sara is the first to consistently say the credit belongs solely to God.

BECOMING OPEN-MINDED

My "Toolchest" of Energy Healers

"The wisdom of the body is responsible for ninety percent of the hope for patients to recover. The body has a super wisdom that is in favor of life, rather than death. This is the power that we depend on for life. All doctors are responsible for letting their patients know of this great force within them."

--Dr. Richard Cabot, former Harvard M.D.

If you told me *before* cancer that I'd lie on a massage table letting a shaman squeeze emotional pain from my body, or enter into a roomful of strangers tapping a plastic doll to ignite the powerful healing possibilities of "Qi energy" from Chinese medicine, I would have thought you were crazy.

I am a smart, well-educated woman, who came from a traditional upbringing and went yearly for physicals with conventional physicians. The "doctor" knows best, I was taught.

Since getting diagnosed, I have learned that doctors know some, but our bodies know a lot more, and our minds have an incredible healing power that we as laypeople can learn to access.

Energy healers can come in many forms—from shamans and acupuncturists to Reiki masters, meditation instructors, and spirit guides. I believe each of these next three energy healers contributed to my changed test results, although no one in conventional medicine can admit that their energy clearing techniques made an impact.

Regardless of whether one believes their efforts on my behalf changed my body, their approaches calmed my mind to the point where I felt heightened moments of joy and bliss that I never experienced before in my life.

Definitions related to "energy as medicine":

"The ultimate approach to healing will be to remove the abnormalities at the subtle-energy level which led to the manifestation of illness in the first place." —Richard Gerber, M.D.

In embracing the increasingly popular "energy as medicine" as a healing tool, it can be helpful to understand at least six key terms:

1.Quantum Physics:

Quantum theory is the theoretical basis of modern **physics** that explains the nature and behavior of matter and energy on the atomic and subatomic level. The nature and behavior of matter and energy at that level is sometimes referred to as **quantum physics** and **quantum** mechanics. —WhatIs.com

According to Wikipedia, *Quantum* is a Latin word that means 'how much.' So a *quantum* of energy is a specific amount of energy. Light sources such as candles or lasers shoot out (or "emit") light in bits called photons. Photons are like packets. Each one has a certain little bit of energy.

For more details, check out:
simple.wikipedia.org/wiki/Quantum_mechanics

www.forbes.com/sites/chadorzel/2015/07/08/six-things-everyone-should-know-about-quantum-physics/#6964606a7d46

2. Epigenetics:

Oversimplified, epigenetics shows how our thoughts, feelings, beliefs, and environments can impact our genes and DNA. Within the last three years, there has been significant data supporting how a change in our thought processes can change our genes. Some in the field believe we are not predestined by our DNA.

For a more detailed explanation, visit:
www.whatisepigenetics.com/fundamentals/

3. Neuroscience:

Neuroscience is the study of the brain and the nervous system, and how the brain's 100 billion nerve cells are born, grow, organize, and connect.

More details of this burgeoning field can be found here:
www.sfn.org/about/about-neuroscience

4. Qi (also spelled Chi) energy:

In Chinese culture, there is a belief that Qi is a force that sustains all life. When blocked or weak, mental or physical consequences can appear, according to Tom Tam, a Chinese healer. On the plus side, this force can be cultivated to empower oneself or heal others through breathing and movement energy work known as Qi Gong.

For a more scientific explanation: wikipedia.org/wiki/Qi

5. Meridian

According to the National Cancer Institute of Cancer, in traditional Chinese medicine, meridians are channels that form a network in the body, through which Qi (vital energy) flows. Blocked Qi causes pain or illness. The flow of Qi is restored by using pressure, needles, suction, or heat at hundreds of specific points along the meridians.

www.cancer.gov/publications/dictionaries/cancer-terms?cdrid=449742

There are 12 main meridians, or invisible channels, throughout the body in which Qi or energy flows. These have no anatomical counterpart in Western medicine. Rather, they relate to processes in the body. Each meridian is a Yin Yang pair, meaning each yin organ is paired with its corresponding yang organ.

6. Chakras

A chakra is a center of energy that helps regulate the body's processes from organ function to the immune system and emotions. There are seven chakras commonly counted, positioned throughout your body, from the base of your spine to the crown of your head. Each chakra has its own vibrational frequency that is depicted through a specific chakra color, and governs specific functions.

To learn more, visit: www.chakras.info

Qi Gong Master, Godfrey

*"For breath is life, and if you breathe well you will
live long on earth." —Sanskrit Proverb*

Breathing New Energy into Life

Just after I learned of my breast cancer diagnosis, but before
having an MRI to confirm the size of my tumor, a dear friend and
client gifted me a one-hour session with Godfrey, a 58-year-old
energetic healer, Reiki and Qi Gong Master, certified massage
therapist, and shaman.

Raw, scared, and willing to try anything to calm myself down, I
accepted the gift with deep gratitude. Openness to new healing
approaches increases for many when confronted head-on with
mortality, I have observed.

Godfrey's first question to me, before I lay down fully clothed on
the massage table, was if I were willing to see the tumor shrink or
go away. "Yes," I nodded, knowing my breast surgeon and her
team would think what I was doing was crazy.

Using a blend of five healing modalities, along with clearing the
room's energy with sage beforehand, Godfrey kept asking if I was
willing to forgive all those who had hurt me in the past. He
repeatedly asked that question, while performing deep tissue
massage, twisting his hands on painful parts of my body to release
old energies and make room for the new healthier energies to
enter, while chanting.

At times, the massage hurt as he came upon a tense spot holding
old energy. The chanting, he explained later, helped raise the
vibration of my body to a higher consciousness, by opening up
blocked meridians in the body. He kept encouraging me to
breathe deeply, exhaling out loudly with sound, to the point
where I would feel exhausted from all this intentional outward
breathing. He then led me through a guided visualization where I

imagined myself in new healing energy under a tree, after walking through an inward journey of letting go through an imagined forest in my mind.

Releasing anger and forgiving others—my parents, my ex-husband, and anyone else who hurt me—continued to be the focus throughout the hour. He kept asking, as he applied pressure to my body, if I was really ready to forgive each person as we listed their names or relationship to me.

At the end of the session, I was calm, peaceful, and felt years younger and lighter. That blissful feeling of open-heartedness remained with me. Driving home, I unexpectedly called my ex-husband whom I had barely spoken to in years, and asked if he would meet with me to do a forgiveness routine together. He agreed.

We used Dr. Hew Len's forgiveness process (shared with me by Lyndra Hearn Antonson, who is now a hospice spiritual counselor), which evolved from the ancient Hawaiian spiritual tradition of Ho'oponopono. It consists in mindfully repeating four simple phrases:

"I'm sorry."

"Please forgive me."

"Thank you."

"I love you."

My ex-husband and I did this process face-to-face on my deck, repeating each statement to one another, and then completing the process by hugging one another.

I did this same forgiveness routine with a friend after a financial deal between us had gone sour. We both cried at the end of our forgiveness statements, and our relationship continues to this day.

Holding in anger and resentment can lead to illness.
Repeatedly practicing forgiveness (for self as well as
others) is one of the most important healing tools.

My MRI, a few days later and to the surprise of my breast surgeon, showed my tumor to be significantly smaller than originally thought, and more specifically that I was in early-stage, not second-stage breast cancer as first believed.

I saw Godfrey again two years later when "a speck" of concern appeared on my other breast. It turned out to be benign.

Godfrey has tracked many other clients who have experienced tumors shrinking or disappearing altogether. He said one man was scheduled for a kidney stone operation, but when the doctor went to operate, there was no stone and the client remained stone-free 10 years later.

Asked why he believes his energy work is so powerful, Godfrey immediately humbled himself. "It is the client, not me, who is responsible for the healings. Those tumors dissolved and shrank because people chose to forgive everything and come back to love," he asserted. "I help you, the client, connect with higher guides and angels to remind you that you are a healer for yourself; all I do is spark the remembrance of that divinity with the lifting of old energy that doesn't serve your highest good and spiral it away with love."

The participation of the client actively engaged for the hour through intentionally loud exhales and visualizations of love and forgiveness is crucial. "You need to do it over and over again, breathe and forgive, until your body thinks and wants to be a divine being of love and light, healthy and sharing your gifts," he said. "Each person is God's child and all I'm doing is reminding them God doesn't want any of his children sick and all we did was forget that we should always be healthy."

Ongoing breath work is key to releasing those old energies. He recommends a daily practice of Qi Gong, which is a conscious energy movement meditation that stimulates self-healing. "Qi" means energy and "Gong" is movement. By connecting breath, intention, and action, a person can strengthen her core and bring balance to the body, mind, and soul, truly feeling connected as one. This type of "unity consciousness" is believed to accelerate healing.

"Remember you are a divine being of love, light, and forgiveness and as you share your unique gifts of creativity with the world you independently unify with higher, infinite consciousness," he noted.

To stay in that mode of "high brain" living, as Godfrey calls it, you need to hear your breath as it is being exhaled.

"The noisier you exhale, the better. You can't think when you hear your sigh," he stressed. "A relaxing sigh opens one to your higher consciousness. If you don't hear your breath, you are still thinking. Practice exhaling more loudly every moment of the day to avoid the lower brain levels of consciousness that feed off pain and drama to keep you alive instead of the infinite light and love of higher consciousness."

Godfrey's energy work has helped people with all sorts of issues beyond physical health, including dealing with grief. He continues to offer one-on-one energy healing sessions, Qi Gong classes, and "Summer of Love Healing Tours" across the country. He shares empowering weekend spring and fall equinox retreats in Sedona, Arizona.

Godfrey resides in Los Angeles and has assisted more than 15,000 people with their self-transformation during his 29 years of energy clearing work in the U.S., Europe, Japan, and Australia.

To learn more about Godfrey's work, contact him directly: godfreylightlove@gmail.com or by phone at 818-438-2888

Michael Wolff – Freedom Within™

"In every culture and in every medical tradition before ours, healing was accomplished by moving energy." —Albert Szent-Györgyi, Nobel Laureate

Opening to infinite love

Three weeks before my scheduled biopsy for the "speck" on my left breast—the second cancer scare—I miraculously made a connection with Michael Wolff, an energy practitioner/healer from the United Kingdom. He reached out to me via LinkedIn and suggested we have a Skype conversation, as we were both in similar professional groups. He had no idea I was writing a book on living from love while healing cancer (as I did not publicly disclose my work-in-progress for fear that I may not get hired— a common fear as I have shared).

Michael believes our thoughts and energetic disconnection— conditioned at birth or in childhood, and continually reinforced by society—contribute to illness. His approach helps clients reach a healthier state of "connection."

By aligning with the creative force of the universe, which Michael described as "the Infinite Love of Source," we can accelerate our healing. In that connected alignment, we are "totally relaxed, centered and at ease," versus operating out of fight-or-flight, which is when our breathing stops, as it does from so many stressors in today's society, he maintained.

> "In neurologically connecting to the whole energy field, one experiences a physical and emotional sense of calm and relaxation."

In awe of the information, I shared with him that I am a cancer survivor. I explained that I was just about to undergo a biopsy for a speck on my "other breast" after insistence by two doctors that I follow through on something my naturopathic doctor and I thought was an imbalance in my body, not a cancerous tumor.

To calm my body and stay aligned with my belief in being cancer-free, Michael offered me a few healing sessions through Skype before my scheduled procedure.

He began by taking an intuitive reading—"muscle testing"—to reveal which chakras in my body were out of balance. Chakras are widely respected, particularly in Ayuverdic medicine, as energy centers that help regulate the body. The seven main chakras include: the root, the sacral, the solar plexus, the heart, the throat, the third eye, and the crown. (To learn more, visit: mindbodygreen.com/0-91/The-7-Chakras-for-Beginners.html)

Through the muscle testing, my solar plexus (the power center on the upper abdomen) and heart chakras showed up as blocked—not surprising given the early childhood traumas I experienced. These early blocks can act as suppressed energy, and attract other similar issues. The result is a weakened immune system, which can make us prone to chronic conditions such as cancer, according to Michael.

My breast cancer, he suggested, may have been directly related to energy blocks I still had in my heart chakra. Had I removed those blocks before my lumpectomy, I may not have needed surgery, he suggested. Yet, in the best-case scenario, by removing them now, I could possibly considerably reduce the chances of, or divert a recurrence of breast cancer altogether, he claimed.

By starting with deep breathing exercises from my lower belly, the key area to commence transformation, Michael led me through four major steps of his process: "Surrender," "Let Go," "Integrate," and "Expansion."

Each step of the way he continued to perform muscle tests to get a benchmark of where I was on a "Map of Consciousness" developed by Dr. David Hawkins and shared in his book, *Power vs. Force.* Zero is the bottom and 1,000 is the top of the scale, which is considered "Buddha" or "Christ consciousness." In mathematical terms, this is a logarithmic scale that expands exponentially, meaning, the highest levels are almost infinitely higher than the very lowest levels.

Michael describes it this way: "Think of a journey that starts in Mumbai, a city on the Indian Ocean, and then travels across the plains and up the foothills all the way to the top of Mount Everest. The bottom of the scale is Mumbai. The top of the scale is the peak of Mount Everest. Base camp on Everest on this scale is the first stage of Enlightenment."

For example, with respect to my own level of harmony, on a scale of 0 to 100, where 100 is total harmony whatever happens in life, and 0 is total disharmony, I calibrated at 78. At the end of my sessions with Michael that total climbed to 100, the top score for that area. On the Hawkins scale, my love rating also climbed to the near 500 desired level.

The third and fourth steps, "Integration" and "Expansion," I continued to do on my own. They involved becoming energetically aware—moment by moment—of the dynamics of resistance and flow. When feeling any emotional resistance, the practice is to:

- Stop and accept.
- Take responsibility for changing oneself.
- BE the Infinite Love of Source.
- Let go in oneself whatever is blocking the flow.

The first stage of connection, where one establishes a connection to their breathing, is like going into a dark room and switching on a light.

"The breath is an energetic connection of life that a child intuitively knows as they breathe naturally from the lower belly," he explained.

"By breathing up (not down as many mistakenly do), you feel the energy come up and spread through all sides and come back down," he said. "It's natural energy. Like a tree, everything flows up and down, expands and contracts. The tree is vertical, everything comes up the trunk, through the leaves to the sky, and flows back down to the roots and back up. And everything from above comes down from the sun, light, through tree, trunk, roots and back up… like a magnetic field around the whole thing."

This breath helps us create a sense of wholeness, by getting out of the head and into the heart, where we often hold our earlier wounds of separation that may have contributed to disease. (Qi Gong master Godfrey had also stressed the need to use breath to get out of the mind and open the body to healing.)

Through the other steps, Michael used powerful creative visualization exercises to help me imagine an emotional pain, or "wounding" as he calls it, being lifted from my body.

"Being fully embodied in connection is so simple but we don't do it," he remarked. "Using sound vibration, and chanting 10 or 15 minutes using AH heart sounds or R like monks do, we identify where the energy is blocked."

Each step of his process helps clients release their earlier core wounds and move up to living in their innate wholeness through:

- acceptance
- forgiveness
- compassion
- unconditional love
- gratitude

Michael's work gave me a heightened sense of awareness, appreciating little things like the hummingbird I saw just as I was about to enter a medical building for that biopsy. I have always loved these tiny little birds. They are a symbol of joy.

I waited four days for the results, continuing to focus on the appearance of the hummingbird I kept seeing. I kept going out each day for long, blissful walks in nature.

My sense of aliveness broadened in nature, with a deep connection to the present that I never before felt so profoundly. Flowers smelled more beautiful, the expanse of the sky seemed like one huge tent of joy above my head, and I "knew" in every cell of my body that I was blessed to experience such exquisite moments of life. I finally realized that *life is in the moments*, and often joy is felt best in the pause of "being" between activities or outcomes.

I finally realized that life is in the moments.

My need for quiet and solitude to connect with God's grace in nature was balanced with "date nights" with my boyfriend as we distracted ourselves from any negative thinking. After allowing myself a few intermittent dark hours of slipping into fright and despair and crying a few worried tears, I intentionally shifted to feelings of joy, recalling all the people I love and who have loved me.

Words of wisdom from others shot forth, like those from my daughter who once shared with me that she enters situations "expecting the best." As a result, she often gets the best. It was my turn to use her thinking, big time, by expecting the best outcome for my biopsy and thoughtfully handpicking a few others who would hold that intention with me.

Then, I recalled the words from my son when I had asked him if he was sad that I was moving cross-country. He'd responded, "I am happy for you. Why would I focus on the sadness?"

Joy is a choice.

Even while waiting for the pathology results from the biopsy, I taught myself to align with that higher vibration of joy, vigilantly challenging any fearful thoughts that cropped up based on having had breast cancer three years prior. I had to train my mind to believe a different outcome was possible this time, particularly as I had been on a unique and comprehensive healing journey.

Hours before getting the call from the doctor, I found myself letting go of such intense focus. Instead, while walking along my favorite lake, I experienced an exquisitely serene sense of surrender and detachment from outcomes. Later that evening, while at a writer's group presentation, my doctor left a voicemail.

After two Skype sessions with Michael, and a clearing technique with Keith Varnum (referenced in the next chapter), my biopsy showed no cancer.

Michael's advice to cancer patients, beyond taking responsibility for their own lives and well-being, is to "Get out of the head and into the heart and feel love (from the belly up) so as not to wobble, stand centered."

For more information about his work, visit:
www.freedomwithin.org.

Keith Varnum

"Energy medicine is the future of all medicine." —Norm Shealy, M.D., founding president of the American Holistic Medical Association

A two-point way of energetically aligning to greater health and well-being

A few weeks after relocating to Arizona, I began searching for spiritual groups where I could connect with like-minded others and be held in high vibrational energy, which I believe is instrumental to healing. From my experiences at The Mind Body Program for Cancer at MGH and Tom Tam's Tong Ren circles, I knew the power of group support. I had often witnessed others feeling instantly better through the more direct exchange of the universal life force of Qi energy.

I came across Keith Varnum's "Find Your Joy" group, which meets twice monthly in Scottsdale and Phoenix, Arizona. His website describes the meeting as a "play shop" that explores the infinite possibilities of transformation through energy healing. "Play" definitely felt like the right word to stay uplifted after my second medical scare. I'd had enough with all the frightful, technical lingo of conventional medicine. Plus, it seemed a lot more fun to heal by playing than by having foreign substances placed in my body.

As I soon discovered, Keith shares 40 years of wisdom he gained from living with Eastern spiritual masters, tribal shamans, Hawaiian Kahunas, and Native American medicine men. Perhaps most profound is his story of overcoming sudden and total blindness at the age of 19, when after traveling the world for a cure, he gave up and picked up a guitar to distract himself from his despair. Suddenly, without explanation, his sight returned. Even the best of medical doctors could not find a logical reason for his new sight. Keith believes it was the joy of playing the musical instrument that shifted his energy and made the spontaneous healing possible.

While in his groups Keith uses a blend of many tools from "brain yoga" to "sacred Tibetan rites," it was his two-point technique from which I experienced many shifts, from new career opportunities to great health.

The first point is the focus of discomfort (what one does not want in life), with the second point being the focus of what one wants (the desired outcome).

In conjunction with the Freedom Within process offered by Michael Wolff, I used this two-point procedure for several days before my biopsy, and Keith also independently from a distance did some two-point procedures for me.

Like I'd learned when I first had surgery for my lumpectomy three years earlier, focusing on the desired outcome and blocking any other thoughts from entering the mind is hugely powerful.

The "two-point" is a quicker, more fun way to shift the focus and bring about new outcomes, particularly when done in a group.

For more information about Keith, his Dream Workshops, and other tools, visit: www.TheDream.com.

Keith's Open-Ended Question Turnaround

Drop into your heart and ask these questions, slowly, one at a time:

1. If I knew how to allow my body to be totally healthy, what would I do?
2. If I knew how to allow my body to be totally healthy, where would my attention go?
3. If I knew how to allow my body to be totally healthy, how would I feel now?
4. If I knew some actions to take to allow my body to be totally healthy, what would they be?
5. If I knew how to allow my body to be totally healthy, what would my life be like?

Then let go and let God (intuition) guide (answer) through clues, messages, and signs. The goal is to add intentions with phrasing that is meaningful and powerful specifically to you and that turn around the unhelpful feeling into a helpful (desired) phrase (prayer, request).

Five Other Healing Tools to Release Emotional Stress and Build Your Immune System

1. Meditating about health on a consistent basis helped me stay aligned with all I learned at The Mind Body Program for Cancer.

I found the Deepak Chopra/Oprah "21-Day Meditation Challenge: Perfect Health" most helpful initially. While meditating each morning, I felt connected to others who were also listening online. Day One began with this introduction by Chopra:

> "There exists in every person a place that is free from disease that never feels pain, that is ageless and never dies. When we journey to this place, limitations we commonly accept cease to exist. They are not even a possibility. This is the place for perfect health. Stepping into this realm, no matter how brief these visits may be, can bring profound transformation and healing. In this state of true mind-body-spirit connection, all previous assumptions about ordinary existence disappear, and we experience a higher truly ideal reality. Sometimes our health is less than perfect, but we need to understand, that is not a permanent state. It is only a snapshot."

> store.chopra.com/21-day-meditation-challenge-perfect-health.html#sm.00000vbkz6bm5kcw4xbd6r0kcxwmv

2. Emotional Freedom Technique (EFT) is a finger-tapping technique, applied to the meridians, to release blocked emotions.

To learn more, visit: eft.mercola.com

www.emofree.com/eft-tutorial/tapping-basics/how-to-do-eft.html

3. Sound Healing - Crystal bowls and gongs... seriously?

One Tuesday night, I had a most blissful evening. I can only liken the contentment to the satisfaction of an orgasm, with my whole body relaxed into a state of surrender and joy. Traumas, dramas, and anxieties of the past and present—including my cancer scare and financial challenges—all felt released from my body.

And I didn't take one drug or mood-altering substance. Instead, I immersed in what my energy healer friend, Keith Varnum, called "a gong bath." This experience entailed an evening gathering of myself and seven other women harmonizing the body, mind, and spirit with Keith using Tibetan singing bowls, custom-made Native American flutes, the gong, and several other sound healing tools.

Years ago, I would have cringed, dismissing this idea as more of that "new age stuff." Listening to sounds from crystal bowls seemed even more frivolous to me for treating medical conditions, particularly more serious ones like cancer. Yet, after confronting my own scary cancer diagnosis, I was willing to try anything that intuitively aligned with my body's innate ability to heal.

Participating in repeated sound healing sessions has allowed me to release a lifetime of pent-up emotions. Sometimes I would cry from the release; other times I felt flu-like symptoms the next day with every bone in my body aching from all the tension I had been holding onto for years. The more often I went, the calmer and happier I became.

Sound healing isn't just for physical health. I gained a greater sense of clarity, awareness, and personal power, and connected more deeply to my essence.

Medical oncologist Dr. Mitchell L. Gaynor, author of *The Healing Power of Sound: Recovering from Life-Threatening Illness Using Sound, Voice and Music,* elaborated on the emotional component of using sound:

> "If we accept that sound is vibration, and we know that vibration touches every part of our physical being, then we understand that sound is 'heard' not all through our ears but through every cell in our body. The sound of our voices, entrained with the sound of the singing bowl, permeates our entire being. Our pulse rate slows and our breath is restored to its natural rhythm. We enter a state of consciousness that allows us to witness our lives from a calmer, more meditative perspective."

Gaynor was highly trained in mainstream medicine and chose to use the medium of sound as an integral part of his approach to healing and wellness. He has seen patients' tumors disappear after using the vibrations from crystal bowls to heal.

"Releasing the past internal blocks is key, for cancer is a wake-up call to our purpose and life calling," he suggested. "It's as if the negative messages received and the traumas experienced since childhood have caused them to become tone-deaf to the true unencumbered voice of their own souls. Odd as it may seem, many of us unconsciously prefer to ignore the summons of our innermost essence. We refuse to emotionally acknowledge our illness and find it difficult to accept healing."

The solution, he maintained, is to stretch out of our comfort zones of the familiar to discover our true, unencumbered selves. For me,

I have been focused on moving beyond "surviving" to thriving for five intentional years. Gaynor's wisdom supports that track.

Even now, after experiencing many miraculous shifts in my state of wellness from attending a variety of sound healing circles using both gongs and crystal bowls, I am met with disbelief and questions of my credibility as a healing agent.

"Don't include that sound healing in your book or you won't be taken seriously," one marketing friend advised. Another colleague distanced from me after I shared that I attend crystal bowl healings regularly. Yet, scientifically the evidence keeps building that sound therapies are at the cutting edge of healing modalities.

In Dr. Gaynor's book, he shares a story of using sound healing for a cancer patient who was dealing with anger and powerlessness over work. He suggested she listen to the vibrations of the crystal bowl, and visualize the source and shape of her fears. She had seen fear as a ball stuck in her throat. "I advised her to play with her own crystal bowl at home daily and she was cancer-free two years later," Dr. Gaynor claimed.

For more information about ordering crystal bowls, visit: www.crystalsingingbowls.com/cms/index.php/dr-gaynor-sound-healing/

In addition to attending sound healing circles regularly, I also experienced blissful states of relaxation through having tuning forks placed directly on specific points on my meridians through a technique known as "Acutonics®" offered by Sunanda Harrell-Stokes, a gifted acupuncturist in Scottsdale, Arizona.

"Sound takes acupuncture to another level," she explained. "When you add sound frequencies directly to the meridians, it is very nurturing and takes only a few minutes to stimulate those points versus 15 to 20 minutes with acupuncture needles."

Harrell-Stokes also customizes the treatments selecting from 50 tuning forks, and using them in combinations to create harmonic intervals based on each client's needs.

Another one of her clients shared: "When Sunanda puts the forks on my body I feel the vibration deep in my bones and I can feel it travel. I feel like I dropped a big burden that I was carrying and I feel much lighter, less worried, and happier."

Most of her acupuncture clients now request the sound healing therapies, using the tuning forks, versus needles, as part of their treatments.

Harrell-Stokes explained the healing power of sound this way:

> "We have all at one time or another experienced a physical trauma from stubbing our toe to some devastating unforeseen accident and everything in between. The one, immediate and automatic response that comes from our corporeal body as a natural and innate response to any type of trauma that impacts the body, mind or emotions is *sound*! Whether that sound is a scream of terror or uncontrollable laughter, the expression of sound is the natural response of our humanity."

Sound is a vibration that is actually a measurable frequency.

In 1900, German theoretical physicist Max Planck revolutionized the field of physics by discovering that energy does not flow evenly but is instead released in discrete packets, which he called "quanta." The nature and behavior of matter and energy at the atomic and subatomic level is referred to as quantum physics and quantum mechanics.

With this new perspective on the behavior of energy and matter, research in physics demonstrated that all matter vibrates and has a resonant frequency.

In his book, *The Seven Secrets of Sound Healing,* Jonathan Goldman says, "We are all unique vibratory beings," and he goes as far to say, "Sound can change the world."

The awareness of infinite possibilities revealed through the continued study of quantum physics and its application to healing through the use of sound, has revealed many discoveries regarding the infinite range of frequencies available to us in nature and particularly through the human voice.

The experiments by Masaru Emoto (youtube.com/tAvzsjcBtx8) show the effects of music and words on water and have demonstrated the interaction of sound on cells.

"There's a consensus of agreement that human beings are made up of 70 percent-plus water," Harrell-Stokes said. "Therefore, it makes sense that we would be dramatically affected as well by the sound effects on water. This explains some of those deep down reactions one has to environmental sounds (hum of the refrigerator, buzz of the computer or a light bulb) including the words one listens to."

For more information on using sound with acupuncture, contact Harrell-Stokes at: sunanda4health@gmail.com.

To learn more about sound healing in general, check out these sites:

- A sample sound healing session at San Diego Cancer Center: youtube.com/bXlHgijQmxw

- More scientific evidence of healing powers of sound:

jbbardot.com/studies-confirm-sound-therapy-heals-arthritis-cancer-tinnitus-autoimmune-disease-and-more-using-vibrational-frequencies/ or youtube.com/bXlHgijQmxw

4. JourneyDance™ – Dancing into love

"Dance and conscious movement bring us back into our bodies, and into the present moment. It is a way of healing the whole person—body, mind, and spirit. It is a path to releasing self-judgment, and moves us to greater self-awareness and self-love." —Corey McLaughlin, life coach and therapeutic movement teacher.

Learning to dance was one of my bucket list items. I wanted to live life experiencing it versus observing it. In the past, I frequently watched my friends joyfully dance as I tensed up on the sidelines, desperately wanting to shed the self-consciousness that came with hiding from a shameful childhood. Occasionally, I would reluctantly and awkwardly dance.

Then, my cancer scare changed how I thought about all my previous dance escapades: No more hiding anywhere for me. Living from love, I was going to claim all of me, even the scared parts that had not been given much freedom to play as a young child. Saying "yes" to new opportunities, and pushing through resistance, became paramount.

Living in real time, knowing that life is not a dress rehearsal, brings me momentum to grasp each moment— which sometimes takes me out of my comfort zone.

The Universe guided me to become more comfortable in my body, bringing me a friend who invited me to a JourneyDance class taught by Corey McLaughlin of Beverly, Massachusetts.

McLaughlin has created a dance studio that feels safe, non-judgmental, and sacred. She helped me gently let my tightly wrapped body loosen and unwind—and as my body became less guarded I rediscovered an ease and playfulness that I had greatly missed.

She herself has loved dance her whole life. "For me dance is absolute joy, and a powerful tool for recovery and healing," she shared. "It quiets all that mental energy and a whole inner space opens up where we find we can express our authentic movement. It invites the heart to soften, and we can connect with ourselves and others."

JourneyDance was developed by Toni Bergins, M.Ed., in 1977. Bergin describes it as, "an empowering journey to self-acceptance and transformation." It is a movement modality that weaves guided sequences and free exploration and helps participants become more fully present and release blocks to inner joy.

The first night I attended McLaughlin's class, she invited our circle of 18 attendees to introduce ourselves and share how we were feeling in that moment. The compassionate and loving environment she created encouraged me to speak honestly.

She made it very clear that we should listen to our own body's wisdom throughout the class. As we began to move and flow to the music we followed imagery in whatever way felt good to us— no right or wrong—as she modeled free-spirited self-expression. There was such freedom in learning that it was about how it felt, not how it looked.

We danced around a fire of our imagination and had a ritual to release negativity into the flames, hollering our "Yes" to life. A point came in the class when we were given scarves to dance with and expand our expression in movement. It felt so freeing to share our heart dances with one another. We returned to the floor to rest our bodies in a blissful state. We later came back to our seated circle to share about what we had experienced.

I didn't expect to feel the way I did, free to be in my body and reconnected to myself as that child who loved to dance. By releasing energy through movement and free expression, JourneyDance helped me shed some of the post-traumatic stress and tension that I'd held in my body from my earlier cancer diagnosis.

"When women get such a diagnosis they often feel negative toward their body, that it has betrayed them," McLaughlin suggested. "They may disconnect from their bodies, and from their sensuality. JourneyDance helps heal the relationship with the body. I hear from breast cancer survivors that it's been helpful to have men in the group also there sharing this experience and bringing their hearts to the dance floor. It is healing to be seen in this compassionate, open-hearted way. A lot of women haven't felt that way in a long time."

McLaughlin is passionate about guiding others to find self-acceptance and love for their bodies through dance and expressive movement. In her classes she sees that people have more energy, gain self-confidence, and simply feel better. This has led her to offer healing dance to people in treatment for serious illness and disease as well as support groups and social service agencies that address postpartum depression and substance abuse recovery.

To learn more about JourneyDance, visit:
www.embodyingsoul.com

5. Panchakarma – Detoxing the body

"Are you ready to dump the past?" Dr. George Savastio, my wise and compassionate naturopathic doctor asked before we commenced the first of five panchakarma treatments. I jokingly responded, "Can you release wrinkles?"

Panchkarma is a cleansing, detoxification, and balancing treatment, successful in treating:

- chronic Lyme disease
- fibromyalgia
- rheumatoid arthritis and other autoimmune diseases
- cancer

It preserves health by removing disease-causing toxins from the body, including residue from pollution, food additives, and our chemically saturated environment, along with the toxins traditionally recognized in Ayurveda as "*ama.*"

According to Dr. Savastio, panchakarma extends beyond other cleansing techniques to remove toxins by reaching beneath the skin to the muscles, joints, and connective tissues where toxic *ama* is lodged. *Ama*, according to Ayurveda, is formed by eating the wrong foods, weak digestive powers, or in response to stress.

"These substances create a stagnation inside the body which blocks the flow of nutrients to tissues and slows the exit of metabolic wastes from tissues," he explained. "By going deeper beneath the skin, panchakarma gives us the ability to more readily reach tissues and joints where the body stores toxins."

Panchakarma is delivered over a relaxing, two-hour period. In contrast to most cleansing therapies, it is frequently a blissful experience.

The four distinct parts of the Ayurveda panchakarma treatment include:

- a deep oil massage (Abhyanga)
- a steady stream of herb-infused warmed oil pouring on the forehead for 30-40 minutes as you relax (Shirodhara)
- a steam bath (Swedana), which literally sweats out the toxins that have been released by the herbal warm oil massage
- an herbal warm oil enema (Basti) for cleansing, nourishing, and lubricating the colon and balancing vata

"My biggest task is to hold the healing space with silence and centered, balanced energy," Dr. Savastio noted. "I also assure the patient is comfortable, feels safe, and that the treatment proceeds properly."

As I was lying on a massage table, naked underneath a sheet, in a darkened room, he began the two-hour cleanse by applying Indian oils, and massaging my feet, to release toxins from the top down. During the steam portion, he sat quietly by, which helped assure me of my safety.

The cleansing of the body had begun with the first treatment, yet the emotional release process was deep.

Session One: November 15, 2013: I left feeling energized, calm, and greasy, as he advised me not to shower until the next day. Leaving the oils on overnight would extend the treatment, he suggested.

I planned nothing for the remainder of the day, except to go home and relax, journal, and stay unplugged from all electronics. In the quiet of letting go of the past, all sorts of new insights came flooding forth. First I felt emotions I was unaware I was carrying, particularly anger for the ways I was not listened to and how I had allowed others to use me or undervalue me.

As I moved through these feelings by journaling, then crying, a new determination emerged as increasing feelings of love and appreciation swelled up within. I fondly remembered my friends from my early days working in public relations as part of a successful team in a fast-growth agency. Those memories came from a different career, a different time in life.

Stepping into the new ways of being I was creating as I released the past, I declared: *I am ready to expand my coaching to teach the self-love I have been embracing, and be valued for my research, expertise, and intuition.*

Instead of being other-centered as I had for a good deal of my life, another question that kept popping up in my quiet time after my first treatment is: "What about me?" It was time to place myself and my needs on the priority list.

Session Two: November 16, 2013: Purged of toxins again, I left this session with diarrhea. Emotionally, I felt very sad, realizing I was still confronting my empty nest syndrome with my son now living with his dad, and my daughter on her own as a college graduate with a new career. Feeling groggy and disgusting from being drenched in oils for the second day, I missed my children and the home life I had as a mother.

In my journal, I wrote: "What am I birthing for me now? A new belief in me and all these old and new connections, and putting my work out in the world and seeing what falls into place and meeting people who can help. I am having conversations with high caliber connections. I am comfortable with high caliber people. I am one of them."

Here are some things I released, whose time had come:

- sense of superiority and determination to do it alone
- my guard
- my judgments
- my perfectionism

My body was healing, but it was time to heal my mind.

The answers are not "out there." I need to be still in myself, stabilize and center my emotions, and accept the gifts of others for what they are, whether an act of service (cooking) or skill (like social networking) or kindness (listening; giving feedback).

What does it feel like to be treasured/cherished/valued? I asked myself.

The response:

Get used to being noticed, be comfortable in your own skin, claim your worth, listen to your gut, take care of you, have fun, and allow someone to have your back.

Session Three: November 17, 2013: Triggered by deceit of people whom I trusted, I knew I had to learn to stay centered and not react. I could feel it, but not lash out. Counting to 10 and going to God, I disengaged from this dysfunctional set-up.

I experienced moments of peace and purity, serenity, knowing my body was clean, free of toxins from panchakarma. I felt lighter, ready for joy and abundance: the joy of connection, loving my new part-time job and its social connections; the joy of listening to music and dancing, being out of my head and into my body; the joy of feeling loved and cared for, and a date taking me out to dinner and a concert; the joy of taking care of my body, and being invited to a yoga class as a gift.

Being lighter, happier, hopeful, and grateful for health and *a new story* of attracting people who have time for me and for whom I can be a priority—with focused attention, not just a convenient companion.

Session Four: November 18, 2013: I left feeling blissful, centered in self, in a deep state of rest and a heightened sense of aliveness. Even colors, such as the tone of my car, seemed more vibrant.

Session Five: November 18, 2013: I felt in deep, deep rest, like a state of nirvana, at peace and grounded in myself. These words came to mind: anxiety-free, calm, determined, in my power, and detached. I felt sensitive, too, sad about the death of my neighbor's son due to heroin overdose, and angry at the manipulation by another to someone for whom I cared.

It was time to develop alligator skin around deceitful people—time to protect me and roar. Grounded in self, and connected to a Higher Power as my partner, I chose to go to God first when something triggers me.

My new beginning was here. I detached and let the past go.

Note: A year later in September 2014, I returned for another panchakarma session, after "a speck" appeared on my left breast. Instead of agreeing right away to the recommended biopsy, I took the advice of Dr. Savastio, who suggested I wait and try to balance my body first. The speck was only showing an imbalance at that point, he said.

Then, he made a profound statement that stuck with me: **"What is the breast? Nurturing and life-giving, and the energy around it would be love, forgiveness, and warmth. That's the energy that would bring health back."**

A month later, I chose to move West with my boyfriend of the time to create a new beginning in a new environment and keep adding love to my life.

To learn more, visit:
elementalmednh.com/shw_services/panchakarma/

REFLECTION

Through my research and personal experience at getting clear test results five years later, I learned in addition to creating a new mindset of unlimited possibilities for health, the following:

- Feel your feelings, then release them.

- Align with the collective unconscious and be around those who believe in and support your body's innate ability to heal. I learned at MGH that those in a mind-body program with others can live up to 2 to 2.5 times longer.

- Find ways to create love and joy in your life. These higher vibrations of consciousness contribute to good health and boost your immune system.

PART THREE:

THE INNER WORK – GOING DEEP FOR LASTING TRANSFORMATION

THE CORE INGREDIENTS OF LASTING CHANGE

"If you're willing to do the mental work, almost anything can be healed." —Louise Hay

As a coach and breast cancer survivor, I have found there are two key pieces of inner "work" one must do to create a new mindset for *living*:

1. **Emotional detox** by releasing negativity from both past conditioning and current life circumstances. To do so, one must feel the lower energy emotions of grief, sadness, anger, and despair, for example, that may have been repressed. Feeling them helps release them and open the way for new more positive emotions of love, joy, and contentment to emerge.

2. **Release limiting subconscious beliefs** that may have contributed as added stressors in your life that weakened the immune system. Once released, one must create new empowering beliefs to move forward from being a victim to a creator of one's life.

This type of work takes great commitment and courage, and is best done with loving support from kind and compassionate people, often trained professionals.

Some transformational leaders believe by continually visualizing positive outcomes—much like an athlete might prepare to win an Olympic event—you can bypass this type of often grueling inner work.

Perhaps, for those who have a stronger inner base of self-love from early childhood, that is the case. Visualization is a powerful

119

tool, especially when you can train yourself to get into the good feeling emotion of the intended end result on a consistent basis.

However, for those who did not receive, through no fault of their own, the core beliefs of self-esteem from the first seven years of life, there is often internal rewiring that must occur.

I always remind clients to be kind and compassionate with themselves when they begin this work. Often they did nothing wrong; they just were not given the basic nurturance in those early formative years that contributed to integrating strong beliefs around feeling worthy or competent.

Our society also continually reminds us, through advertising, to look for and want more externally to feel good enough and worthy, rather than know our intrinsic value "as is."

It may seem easier (and less time-consuming than the vigilance required to rewire the brain) to rely on external sources for a "cure." Medications, nutritional supplements, and treatments can bring the body back in balance or remove, shrink, or prevent a tumor from recurring.

> ### The Guest House
>
> *"This being human is a guest house. Every morning a new arrival.*
>
> *A joy, a depression, a meanness, some momentary awareness comes as an unexpected visitor.*
>
> *Welcome and entertain them all! Even if they are a crowd of sorrows, who violently sweep your house empty of its furniture, still treat each guest honorably. He may be clearing you out for some new delight.*
>
> *The dark thought, the shame, the malice, meet them at the door laughing and invite them in.*
>
> *Be grateful for whatever comes, because each has been sent as a guide from beyond."*
>
> *—Rumi*

Yet, to find the underlying causes of what brought a disease like cancer on, it helps to dig a little deeper, particularly if you weren't pre-disposed through genetics. Even if you have some genetic disposition, there are many in neuroscience who now believe you can change your DNA, including Dr. Bruce Lipton, who I have referenced for his work around epigenetics.

It has been my personal experience in healing my childhood, and witnessing hundreds of clients do the same, the emotional detox and belief change processes often help elevate the mind and body to optimal states of health and well-being. Proper nutrition and exercise, along with establishing a strong spiritual base, also help accelerate the healing process.

The Scary Part

You must face some darkness to reach the light.

Spiritual leader and author Joyce Rupp articulates this journey within so eloquently in her book, *Little Pieces of Light: Darkness and Personal Growth*:

> *"We always try to have a balance—to enter freely into the waiting room of darkness and yet not gorge ourselves on the pain and discomfort. We have probably met people who wear their woes and old hurts like a breastplate of self-importance. It's their way of drawing attention to themselves, of deriving some long-sought human care and compassion, or of meeting some other deep need.*
>
> *The stirrings in the tomb of darkness are the whispers of our soul, urging us to move toward a place we have not been before. We may be pushed to make changes we would otherwise never have considered. We may be forced to look at hidden wounds and inner issues we were always able to shove aside. We may be led to appreciate life and our gifts at a more extensive and deeper level. Usually the womb of darkness provides a catalyst for creativity and a full relationship with the Holy One. Always it is a time for trust in the transformative process and for faith that something worthwhile may be gained by our waiting in the dark."*

No one is exempt from negative conditioning; it is part of our inheritance of the human condition, according to Dr. David Hawkins in his book, *Letting Go: The Pathway of Surrender*. He writes:

> "Finding out what needs to be cleaned up is simple and easy. Just look at what you would not want others to know about you and begin to surrender it."

Learning to forgive (both ourselves and others), and releasing guilt are two of the most healing processes for surrender, Dr.

Hawkins maintains. Guilt only results in self-punishment, allowing others to criticize, belittle, and invalidate us, he notes in his book.

EMOTIONAL DETOX YOUR BODY:

Emotions count, big-time: "Your Issues in Your Tissues"

"Emotion is just energy in motion, so you have to allow it to move. When you suppress your emotions and do not allow them to move through expressing them, this will create physical imbalances, and you now have issues in the tissues." —*Dr. Mahdi Brown*

By the time I arrived at Dr. Mahdi Brown's lecture, "Your Issues in Your Tissues," three years after my cancer diagnosis, there was no doubt that I was being divinely guided in my healing and writing journey.

Beyond having healing sessions gifted to me, I continued serendipitously to meet the "right" person for the message I needed to hear. At the last minute a friend changed her plans with me and suggested we go hear Dr. Mahdi, as he likes to be called, speak.

Dr. Mahdi is a naturopathic doctor, professor, life coach, and author.

Dr. Mahdi's energy exudes a love and zest for life so powerful you feel your own vibration instantly rise just by being in his presence. Being with him is like "one-stop" shopping, as his breadth of expertise from the scientific, nutritional, and medical to the psychological and spiritual components of health is so comprehensive.

What I wasn't prepared for was finally, and in great depth, hearing words from a doctor that validated my own intuitive prompting early on that emotions, and spiritual connection to the love that we innately are, contribute greatly to our health.

Whew! I felt more empowered than ever. My self-crafted beliefs about the healing journey had even more scientific back-up than I originally intuited! I was not crazy in the way some in conventional medicine seemed to judge me for undertaking an alternative route.

I could barely stay seated as each word Dr. Mahdi uttered inspired me even more to stay on the path I had chosen and to share all I learned about our body's innate ability to heal.

Cancer is a state of health based on our internal and external environments.

"The body is a reflection of the consciousness that is occupying the space," Dr. Mahdi claimed at the beginning of his lecture. "The body is designed to always seek homeostasis [balance/health]. It is constantly adapting itself to this end based on the environment in which it finds itself. Therefore, diabetes, cancer, and any so-called dis-ease is a state of health based on the environment in which the body is currently finding itself. When you shift the so-called dis-ease environment internally—physically, mentally, emotionally, spiritually—and externally, the body will adapt itself to accommodate the new environment and adjust its state of homeostatic expression. In essence, the body is able to experience a higher state of homeostasis and health, and you heal."

Dr. Mahdi further asserted that the body is always seeking to maintain balance for the highest expression of energy and life that it can. "Your body is here to serve you," he said. "It's not your enemy. The body by design only seeks health."

In fact, emotions are the link to the mind-body connection. Love, in particular, is "nutrition for the brain and every other cell in your body," according to Dr. Mahdi.

Most of us are seeking to feel good. Someone with a high self-image, for example, wakes up excited and enthused. She has great expectations for her day. Her excitement and enthusiasm affords her energy and vitality throughout the day. She is a joy to be around and her energy can be infectious. Dr. Mahdi suggested to ask yourself: When you feel most *alive*, what are you doing in life?

Like I learned from my training with Dr. Dispenza, Dr. Mahdi also believes that to raise one's self-image and correlating feelings of self-love, a person needs to create a new image of self through asking and imagining: *What if you could be the greatest version of yourself in this moment, how would you feel, look, and be right now?*

Your body must reflect this new imagined state of self in energy and vitality. Therefore, you must renew your body as you renew your mind. This is done through eating nutrient-dense, cleansing foods that alkalize the body, he claimed. Your body will then have the ability to rid itself of toxins that are not serving it and causing dis-ease.

The number one way to detoxify emotions that are standing in the way of feeling good and living in optimal health is to express ourselves and speak our truths, he said, noting that women tend to hold their unresolved mental and emotional traumas in the breast tissue and reproductive tissues.

"When the sacred feminine essence of who they are as women is compromised, denied, or rejected, it shows up in these tissues," Dr. Mahdi said. "Heavy, painful menstruation is a sign of the body being overly burdened with toxins chemically, mentally, and emotionally. In an ideal world, women would take that week off. It's sacred time. It's creative energy."

Finding our voice, and authentically expressing self, is perhaps one of the most powerful healing tools. He believes we are all given three gifts: a mind and heart to guide us on what to do, and a voice to express who we are on this planet. "Through your voice, you are given the ability to communicate and find a healthy way to express your feelings and thoughts."

Addressing the high-stress mode of fight-or-flight is also important in bringing the body back to balance. Learning to be still, and present, can eliminate ninety percent of stress, Dr. Mahdi shared.

Fight-or-flight is an anxious state, a physiological reaction to a perceived threat. "The body's cells start to isolate, then go into protective mode, which can lead to disease," he said, adding, "When you shift out of fight-or-flight, the body will feel it. True healing does not simply alter a person's body. It alters the person's inner self."

In a follow-up interview with Dr. Mahdi a few weeks after his lecture, he elaborated even further on the emotional power of self-love as a major contributor to health.

"We heal by being thankful and in love and fully accepting of who we are, regardless of our circumstances," he said. "We have the ability to create a whole new reality by letting go of preconceived notions, shame, or guilt toward ourselves. From a place of thankfulness and self-forgiveness, we are able to let go of condemnation and judgment of what we have experienced in life so far. This mental and emotional releasing will translate into biochemical and physiological expression within the body that are able to heal."

Claiming our worthiness and taking actions to support it directly impacts health.

"Prolonged self-hate and judgment and being ashamed of who we are and what we are in life has no choice but to express itself in tissues," he said. "When you take a step back and say, 'OK, I matter enough to make the changes,' and let go of what is no longer serving you intuitively, you can heal naturally."

The most important shift can occur by making a life-or-death choice and then staking a claim on the declaration of choosing to live.

Dr. Mahdi calls this choice 'a healing decision' around self-love.

"Self-love is the foundation of who we are and how we perceive the self, which determines the choices we make," he said. "The biggest detriment to healing is a person's inability to make a healing decision of self-value, self-worth, getting healthy, and living in vibrant health. Many hold to the story of illness, hold the label of being sick, and they do not recognize the body by design is always thinking health."

Upon hearing a diagnosis or facing an illness, Dr. Mahdi asks his clients the following questions:

- **Do you really want to be here?**
- **Do you want to live?**
- **What do you want for your life?**
- **Is there something more still for you to do?**

In my healing circles I have heard from many others whose tumors completely disappeared when they intentionally made a declaration to themselves that they were choosing to live versus die.

"When we choose life, life chooses us, and we're afforded more life," Dr. Mahdi maintained. "Observe a baby. It's always choosing life, letting the Universe know it's here, so present and full of life."

Stay faithful to that vision, with all thoughts focused on choosing life.

"All other options are null and void," he urges clients to believe. "It's now about healing and about life, and with that mindset and vision, the healing will come about."

Anyone newly diagnosed with an illness needs to know that the healing power resides within each patient, he said, adding:

"Within the body, every living creature on this planet has the code of healing in it. Based on being present with ourselves, we can be guided to what is needed for healing, regeneration, and from the current state of how to show up in more vibrant health."

128

Reframing negative events as high growth opportunities versus viewing them from a victim mentality also can help one heal. By embracing forgiveness and creating thoughts of gratitude, one can shift from things happening *to* them, to circumstances occurring *for* them, he explained.

"The hard truth is for anyone to know that he or she has to take responsibility for his or her life," he said. "You can't blame anyone or any circumstances."

Finding one's life purpose also can help a person heal, he said, noting that pathology is a study of your path. "You develop a pathology when you are no longer aligned with your highest purpose and path so the pathology will sound an alarm to stop you," he explained. "Now, you have an opportunity to make a new choice and align with the highest expression and path. Disease can hold a space for you to rise up, shift, and carry out the unique curriculum and calling of your soul."

> The spiritual significance of knowing one's innate power, and choosing life, is embracing this thought, according to Dr. Mahdi:
>
> "You are a unique expression that life has never witnessed before, nor will it witness again once you're gone. We are all divine. Your life is your spiritual practice."

Dr. Mahdi's Tips for
Staying Physically Healthy

- Vitamins are needed to replace nutrients lacking in our foods today. He frequently recommends: high quality multi-vitamins, B-complex, Vitamin C, and fish oils that support every system in the body. The right dosages depend on each individual and should not be self-prescribed.
- Get at least seven hours of sound sleep per night, as the body can only heal itself when at rest. Deep meditation can also help produce a restful state. Without giving the mind and body time to rest, the nervous system becomes impaired which can affect the whole body.
- Eat organic, nutrient-dense foods in their most wholesome state, directly from the earth when possible. Have something "green" every day. The chlorophyll in leafy greens is especially helpful for cleaning and building new blood.
- Detoxify the body with seasonal cleanses.
- Ensure you are properly hydrated, as water is the substance of life. A person should drink at least half of their body weight in ounces of purified or spring water a day.
- Move your body, which is its main purpose for being here. The ideal baseline is 30 minutes a day beyond the first signs of perspiration. Movement can be any activity from yoga, dance, or walking to a gym workout or even play on the beach.
- Find your mission, purpose, and goals, to give your brain a vision upon which to focus.
- Create a mind based on love and make the healing decision to choose life.

TRAINING THE MIND TO HEAL THE BODY

Words matter – focus on what you want

By focusing each day on the following list of empowering words, emotions can be elevated.

Elevated emotions plus clear intentions help create a new mindset for living, Dr. Dispenza and others taught me in my healing journey. A more joyful mindset can impact the health of our cells, helping build a stronger immune system.

Here is the list of words I have collected to help shift my consciousness into a greater state of well-being:

Empowering Words

Some words that lift you to a love-based consciousness:

Healthy	Honored	Enthused
Vibrant	Respected	Joyful
Worthy	Appreciated	Cherished
Loving	Validated	Aligned
Lovable	Nurtured	Excited
Loved	Nurturing	Validated
Wanted	Supported	Grateful
Accepted	Connected	Contented
Celebrated	Trusting	Empowered

To shift energy using these empowering words, it helps to create a new list of what you want (versus focusing on what you don't want).

These "wants" give energy a new area in which to flow:

- Spend time each day dreaming about and imagining yourself living in the new want.
- Script the health outcome you want.
- Expect new results.
- Talk tenderly and lovingly to yourself every day.
- Focus more on FEELING the high vibration emotion, versus on all the "doing" of the day.
- Watch for clues, and jot down evidence of the new "want" arriving.

Environments matter – find your happy place

"There is no need to go to India or anywhere else to find peace. You will find that deep place of silence right in your room, your garden, or even your bathtub." —Elisabeth Kubler-Ross

A few people have been worried about me starting over again, alone in Arizona after the relationship that brought me here ended. I had a few panic moments myself thinking I should return East, but then something larger than my ego self told me to stay.

To begin with, the ease with which my new apartment "appeared" seemed rather miraculous. One day while walking, instead of taking my normal route by the lake, I veered off to buy a cup of coffee, something I rarely drink these days. Walking back home, I noticed an "apartment for rent" sign on the sidewalk by one of my favorite lakeside complexes.

Thinking I could never afford to live there as I had priced nearby rentals before, I called the listed number anyway. The kind man who answered the phone informed me the unit he and his wife owned was available for lease now (two months before I was planning to move), and at a slightly higher cost than I was willing to pay. He suggested he could perhaps hold the unit for two months if it seemed a match for me.

I agreed to meet him at the unit the following morning. When I walked in, I had to hold my breath for a dream was manifesting before my eyes. The unit was completely furnished in exactly my taste, to the point that the living room rug was the exact same rug I once had in my office studio back East. The high-top kitchen chairs were the exact same ones I had in one of my former kitchens.

Moreover, the apartment had just been gutted and renovated with exquisite taste. I was so focused on completing this book that the last thing I wanted to do was upgrade or decorate a home. What a gift!

Before making a decision, I asked him (and his wife who later showed up), if I could sit alone in the apartment for a few minutes to get a feel for it. They agreed and moved outside to the deck.

I sat in the living room and closed my eyes, barely able to contain myself. Being in this home felt like being wrapped in a big hug, as one of my writer friends later described it.

Such huge feelings of gratitude welled up inside for I had found the perfect writing nest, a quiet corner unit with a soothing fountain beneath the deck where I knew I would write many, many words.

I told the landlord I had to think about it for a few hours, as I wasn't prepared to move so quickly or pay that much. He offered my desired move date and we negotiated the rent.

As he walked me to the entrance gate outside, he asked what I was writing. I told him of this book, not sure if he would still rent to me as some people fear the cancer word, but I chose to risk honesty nonetheless. It turned out that he, too, is a cancer survivor. That commonality felt like another assurance that this was the right place for me.

The day I moved in six weeks later, a bottle of wine and card from my landlord were waiting for me. The card read: "Life holds so many happy little moments just waiting to be noticed." How appropriate for someone like me who has learned post cancer that life is truly in the moments, and often the simple ones are the richest.

The initial lonely days are slowly evolving into a sacred quietness, where I kindly talk to God and myself as I pace this new beginning in loving, compassionate ways.

Loving myself means not "wronging" or letting others wrong me for getting placed in this new home of yet another rebirth.

I am in a grand surrender, and playing witness to my life, observing what roles I have played in what has not worked, and how I am being guided forth in new ways.

THE BELIEF WORK

Understanding "Our Internal Operating System"

"Positive thoughts have a profound effect on behavior and genes, but only when they are in harmony with subconscious programming... When it comes to sheer neurological processing abilities, the subconscious mind is millions of times more powerful than the conscious mind." —Bruce Lipton, Ph.D., *The Biology of Belief/Change*

"Almost universally, the experiences that cause people to feel stuck have roots in what are considered negative beliefs created early in life. And it's precisely because they are subconscious that it's often difficult for us to see them in ourselves... Ninety percent or more of our daily actions are responses that come from the reservoir of information we accumulated during the first seven years of life... The reality is that most of us learned our subconscious habits in an environment that was a mixed bag." —Gregg Braden, *The Spontaneous Healing of Belief*

In the following pages, I share intimate glimpses in ways I learned to rewire old beliefs or integrate new ones throughout my healing journey.

Please Note:

Owning the new beliefs we want to live from is a two-fold process. First we have to become conscious of the hidden, false beliefs that no longer serve us. Then, we have to claim the new belief and consistently act on it (it is best to take an action on the new belief within 24 hours). Changing a belief requires vigilance to overtake the hard-wiring of early conditioning. Repeat it out loud upon waking and again five minutes before you go to bed each evening (the best times to download new information in the subconscious). Writing the belief down also helps integrate it and create a new neural pathway in the brain. Focus on the new outcome, not the past.

There can often be moments of sharp contrast between the old way of seeing ourselves and the new possibility, which can create angst. In this triggered moment of choice, we get to decide if it is too painful to continue living from the old belief even though it can be scary to step into the unknown of the new belief.

Raising the bar for our lives to a new way of being is not a simple process. Our ego tries to keep us in the familiar. To learn more about this dynamic at the subconscious level, I often recommend *The Big Leap: Conquer Your Hidden Fear and Take Your Life to the Next Level* by Gay Hendricks, Ph.D. Hendricks explains in great detail ways we subconsciously sabotage change for the better.

Here is an example of acting in new ways: Right after I wrote about claiming my power, in a subsequent chapter, I got to test it out in real life to see if I had really integrated knowing I am an internally powerful woman. I became aware of a situation in which I was not paid the same amount for my work as other colleagues. Rather than keep my feelings simmering within, I spoke up. I centered within first, choosing to respond versus react.

Then, when I did not feel fully heard or seen in the discovery of the rate disparity, I calmly walked away, not sure I'd still have my job, but knowing I had to honor myself in that moment regardless.

The choice to express my shock was not so much about the dollar value of the money, but about knowing and claiming my value. My request for more money was heard and honored. I have had to make similar decisions consistently through this process of reinvention.

Claiming our value does not necessarily mean aggressively asking for what we want. Sometimes it means quietly saying "no" to ways others treat us that are unacceptable, and simply standing in our own strength of the conviction that we deserve more respect.

"Owning our story can be hard but not nearly as difficult as spending our lives running from it. Embracing our vulnerabilities is risky but not nearly as dangerous as giving up on love and belonging and joy—the experiences that make us the most vulnerable. Only when we are brave enough to explore the darkness will we discover the infinite power of our light."

—Brené Brown, *The Gifts of Imperfection: Let Go of Who You Think You're Supposed to Be and Embrace Who You Are*

Six Core Beliefs of Healthy Self-Esteem

1. I allow myself to know I am lovable.

2. I allow myself to know I matter.

3. I allow myself to know I have value because I exist.

4. I allow myself to know I am worthwhile.

5. I allow myself to know I can handle my self and my environment with competence.

6. I allow myself to know I have something of value to offer others.

From *Your Child's Self-Esteem,* by Dorothy Corkille Briggs

A CORE BELIEF OF SELF-ESTEEM

"Life becomes more dynamic when my beliefs are dynamic." —Deepak Chopra

Glimpse #1: I AM ENOUGH

Knowing "I am enough" is a core belief to healthy self-esteem. Yet, many struggle with it, including superstars like the former Whitney Houston as described in a blog I wrote after her death (supportmatters.com/knowing-you-are-enough). During an interview with Diane Sawyer, Houston said she never felt "enough" to perform with Kevin Costner in the movie, *The Body Guard.* Her fame, beauty, and talent could not give her the sense of greatness she had been unable to claim for herself.

In healing cancer, I repeatedly chose to claim "I am enough," versus see myself as a less than desirable woman because I had a scarred breast. No victim story would be created around this health challenge, I vowed.

Increasingly, I began to see that the courage to follow the path I chose had filled me up, rather than taken away from the essence of who I am. I had new levels of depth and wisdom from many hours spent in contemplation.

Still, remnants of inadequacy popped up now and then, particularly around my health choices. One day, after a long, intense day of writing at a local restaurant, I accepted and savored every bite of the complimentary bread pudding dessert offered me.

The next morning, waking up at 5 a.m. to hike with a friend, I recalled how healthy my diet and lifestyle have become since being diagnosed with cancer. I start each day with my own homemade green shake, a walk or hike, yoga, meditation, and journaling. I have slowed way down, often enjoying many moments of just "being" versus running around doing.

Still, eating that decadent bread pudding dessert made me consider that I had not done enough to stay clean post cancer. Sugar is a no-no as it can be a magnet for cancer cells. Yet, when I ate the more rigorous diet without wheat, sugar, or dairy upon first getting diagnosed, I looked anorexic and felt deprived.

Joyful living is part of the commitment to the new self I am reinventing. Finding the balance of doing enough to stay healthy while also enjoying life's occasional splurge is a continual challenge.

"You must be strict on this diet. There is no variation allowed," a doctor advised, when I told her of my choice to decline radiation. Today, I forgave myself and told myself *I am enough*, whether I abided by the rules or not. Quality of life matters, and yes, I feel much better when I eat healthy, but it was pure fun to sneak in an indulgent treat. Isn't fun good for us, too?*

Dr. David Hawkins has said that when one lives in the higher love state of 500 or above on his scale of consciousness, dietary restrictions are not necessary. The elevated emotions are more healing than the foods we eat.

Glimpse #2: I AM POWERFUL

I have the ability to connect with the power of my mind to heal my body.

"Many of us have a secret or unconscious death wish," Godfrey, my early energy healer once told me. At first that thought seemed incredulous, but then I came across others who, in moments of despair, shared they felt that dying would be better than living.

I know people who had spontaneous healings of cancer when they made a conscious decision to live after carefully reviewing whether they were ready to die. Somewhere in that choice I suspect, if they are anything like me, they also had to declare their value independent of what others think of them.

Sure, I have helped hundreds of people over the years shift their lives in more joyful, meaningful ways, and received great satisfaction from that work. Yet, I couldn't fix past mistakes and betrayals that led to financial chaos. I felt powerless. Choices made long ago (when I had much lower self-esteem), based on giving to others at the expense of myself, still had consequences in my life decades later.

It was in that sense of powerlessness, and leaning in and feeling it, that I had the most significant emotional healing of my life.

How could I change the story, so I could keep my health back on track, my joy for life magnified, and avoid financial disaster based on past trauma?

I spent a good deal of a year alone sending out resumes, networking, then walking, writing, and praying. For two months I disengaged from most of the world, meditating two, three, and even sometimes four hours a day.

Once, in the midst of my self-imposed retreat, I awoke and sobbed for hours. I couldn't believe I had so many tears left. Everyone close to me had heard my tales of woe, many, many times of how hard I tried to turn it around. It was such an old story by now. The block could not be about money, or lack thereof. Nothing made sense. Something bigger was at play here.

Then, with a great deal of self-love, compassion, and forgiveness, I got the "aha." Deep, deep within me, I had a belief that I was powerless. As a young girl, I couldn't fix my mom, or make her better or happier, no matter how hard I tried. Her brain disease got the best of her, and I took it on as my own failure. Whatever I did (performing in any way I could to please her, from getting straight A's to always being "good") made no difference in her health or happiness.

Tips

- Choose to live. Declare that commitment.

- Determine how you will live that life in an empowering way by asking: If I knew I were a truly powerful person, what choices would I make in my life today, tomorrow, next week?

- To increase your sense of value and power, get quiet and ask: Is there is a part of me longing for expression that has not been brought forth or honored yet?

Damn, I tried so hard to help her and when I could not, then I tried hard to win the approval of others through external accomplishments.

Sadly, without a role model of competency, I also developed an inner sense of helplessness and neediness, never quite sure I was doing anything right. I attracted many rescuers along the way to "help me," a pattern of behavior that creates co-dependency, not the joy of self-reliance and self-sufficiency.

My cancer healing journey of dedicating myself to honor the innate wisdom of my body required I change that pattern. I couldn't defer this task to someone else. I needed to rescue me, and integrating higher levels of self-esteem was important.

In the process of that discovery, I learned true power doesn't come from the outside world. It comes from within. To know myself as an *innately* powerful woman for the first time in my life, I had to do five things:

1. Grieve all those years of trying so hard and assuming responsibilities that were never mine to begin with. Sitting with the pain that I had repressed for a lifetime took a full day of crying, followed by a few unsettling days as I let go of old patterns of "pushing" that no longer served me.

2. Connect to God, or a Higher Power and continue building faith by seeing, even when I felt I couldn't support myself, that I was being "carried." So many friends and acquaintances helped along the way. I lost everything that the outer world viewed as success. My pride was crushed, but my creativity got ignited.

3. Claim the power that "I Am." Writing is a God-given talent bestowed upon me. Completing this book was no longer about me or ego-satisfaction. Rather, I started seeing it would be selfish not to share with others at diagnosis what it took me five years to learn and integrate.

4. Know I am valuable 'as-is,' for just being, regardless of the outcome of a project, or any other task I initiate. During the times I had the least amount of money I often made some of the richest connections of my life. Being transparent, vulnerable, and genuine is more valuable than the tally of our financial accounts.

5. Make a choice to *thrive*, not just survive, by fully expressing the essence of who I am.

Letting go of what it looks and feels like

Releasing the old, victim-based, driven me was not a smooth transition. Yet, the discomfort and angst of letting go of past ways opened my heart and mind for new levels of joy. Elevated emotions help keep us healthy, as Doctors Hawkins and Dispenza claim.

Gaining a sense of power is particularly important to anyone newly diagnosed. The more involved a patient is in his or her own care and creating an optimist attitude the more they can impact their longevity.

Glimpse #3: I ALLOW MYSELF TO KNOW I AM WANTED

Even though I felt rejected or betrayed in my life by those I loved—and even now by the medical community that cannot validate my choices—it wasn't until four years after reinventing myself post cancer that I discovered a very powerful word for creating shifts in my life and with my clients: *Wanted*.

For decades before, I helped clients clear limiting beliefs and integrate new ones around their lovability. This new word, which came to me when I was working diligently to release negativity from my own past, seemed to have more impact. Underneath my despair from early life conditioning, I realized I had an underlying expectation and belief that those I loved would reject me.

I bless and forgive my mother every day for I cannot fathom the terror of living with a disease like schizophrenia. Still, her inability to be present in the nurturing way every child deserves left me subconsciously feeling rejected. Attracting people who withdraw when I expressed a need felt "normal" having watched my mother in catatonic states for years. Life was about her, and keeping her calm.

To heal that wound brought to consciousness in my process of reinvention, I started telling myself "I Am Wanted." Then, I would journal on what it felt like to be wanted. Layers and layers of feeling used, abused, neglected, bullied, humiliated, ignored, and raged upon came forth. Tears followed, observing all those who loved me when I did something for them, but couldn't handle when I wasn't the strong, supportive person with needs of my own. "Too emotional" is the defense they would use. Being made to feel wrong was a chronic pattern of life.

Even the day I got my suspicion-of-cancer-diagnosis after my mammogram, I stared across at the stoic, cold face of the radiologist incredulous that not one word of warmth or comfort was offered by him as I sat there crying. He was a male version of my mom, except she had the excuse of being heavily medicated to calm the nerves within her chaotic body.

Silence is not golden; it can be excruciatingly painful when someone is in need of love and reassurance.

I have since learned, when triggered by the person in front of me, to pace myself and not react before centering within to respond with as much love and personal responsibility as I can. Love is, after all, a discipline—knowing which part I play in the engagement, and which part comes from the past or another's "story."

Equally important, when I don't feel wanted now, is to self-soothe, speaking as lovingly as possible, giving myself the gentle and compassionate nurturance I didn't receive in my cravings for kindness. Another person's inability to be present is not a reflection of me; rather it is his or her own wounds to heal.

To move forward in self-love and higher consciousness, I need to keep cherishing myself, whether someone validates my desirability or not.

Coincidentally, weeks after writing this chapter, my friend lent me her Loving Kindness Meditation. These profound words at the introduction of the CD have become my new focus: *"Kindness heals; judgment wounds."* Directing those thoughts to myself (and others) has become increasingly important as I teach the cells within my body that they are loved and cared for by a nurturing presence.

The life of a cancer survivor can feel lonely, as few (me included) want to talk about the dreadful disease. The life of a writer, with all its blissful freedom to express oneself from the depths within, can also feel lonely. Rejection slips are the normal part of doing business in my field.

Still, I know the *feeling of being wanted*, and associating with that, can change outcomes. Being "wanted" is another reason for living—finding the community that embraces me is an ongoing part of my journey.

I have set up a new expectation and am aligning with infinite possibilities of how the Universe will validate my inner knowing and belief of my value.

In the meantime, I'm going to continue cherishing myself. Who knows? Feeling wanted may impact my longevity, and give me even more of a reason to *Choose Life*!

Tips

- If you knew you were wanted, what would your life look like?
- How can you "want" yourself and validate all your gifts and talents?

Additional resources for integrating a sense of love and compassion to help instill the belief of being wanted can be found in *Self-Compassion* by Kristin Neff, Ph.D.

Glimpse #4: I MATTER

Choose to become visible. Place yourself in situations where you are seen, heard, and validated.

As noted previously, sometimes when we're shifting a limiting, subconscious belief to a more powerful and healthy one, contrasts appear. Feeling the pain of the unwanted feeling or situation can help you claim more fervently the new desire you seek to manifest.

There are some in Law of Attraction communities focused more intently on outcomes who would disagree with this approach, but I align with the work of Dr. David Hawkins and the healing miracles he has initiated and witnessed. He believes it is in letting go of negative emotions by feeling them, without judgment, that we move forward.

When we're committing to a new goal, sometimes we must review the internal blocks that stopped us from achieving it before, and intentionally choose to focus differently for new success. Often those blocks are based on subconscious beliefs created during the first seven years of life, and have little to do with our current intellectual capacity or circumstances.

Plunging into the depths of my being, with intent to clear negativity from my soul, I kept crossing paths with narcissists (like my mom, whose illness helped her become the center of attention with others' needs surpassed). Like many others subconsciously trained to give to others at the expense of themselves (which includes a lot of people in the helping professions), I got highly triggered.

Sure there was a bit of "mirror, mirror on the wall" reflection showing me where I had been too self-absorbed from dramas around sadness and despair of years past. Yet, digging deep, the pain of these new encounters ignited all the ways I had felt invisible from not being seen, heard, and validated in loving, nurturing, and compassionate ways from early conditioning.

In owning further personal responsibility for healing the wound from the false, negative belief that I don't matter, I consistently continue to choose one or more of the following seven options to integrate the healthier new belief of mattering:

- Speak up when someone talks without listening to what I have to say.

- Remove myself from the situation, and center within, acknowledging myself in the ways I hoped someone or some external event would provide.

- Bless the self-absorbed person in front of me, seeing with compassion his or her unmet need for attention.

- Forgive myself for the times I have been self-absorbed during "needy" moments in life, when I felt I was tossed a curveball I couldn't handle and needed someone to listen for hours on end.

- Seek out others aligned with reciprocally sharing.

- Instill the belief that *I Matter*, and track evidence daily of being supported in that stronger sense of self.

- Risk being more visible.

Being a patient (whether you have cancer or some other illness) can ignite painful feelings of invisibility and feeling like you don't matter. Insurance-induced mandates for the number of patients per day or hour physicians must tend to do not leave much time for us to be seen, heard, and supported on all the levels that contribute to good health—emotional, physical, mental, and spiritual. Sadly, many doctors I know feel the same pain of their powerlessness in the bureaucratic system that leaves them little time to give the type of care their patients need and deserve.

Instead of being victims, we must build our own teams of support people who have the time to help lovingly nurture us back to good health.

Moving forward, with an innate sense of knowing you matter, also means risking being more visible in many other ways outside your healing journey.

The inner time of reflection and integration is necessary as a respite to bridge the gap between the old and new ways of being.

Yet, allowing yourself to be seen on a stage, in a classroom, at a meeting, working with the public, or in a relationship, is another way of claiming *I Matter*. Visibility heals; isolation does not.

If you knew you mattered, what new choices would you make for your health and well-being?

Glimpse #5: I AM WORTHY

As I progressed on rewiring my own brain through the five-year healing journey detailed in this book, I became more adamant about claiming my worthiness. I continually raised the bar by asking for what I wanted, experimenting more with choices, taking greater risks, and visualizing a far bigger picture of my future than I had in the past.

Now, my focus is on knowing I am worthy of joy, peace, contentment, and fulfillment—moving beyond surviving to thriving, to a new life story.

Paradoxically, we are all born worthy. It is not something we need to "do" or prove—a mistake I made earlier in life by looking at my achievements to define me. Yet, we can get blocked from feeling and acting on that innate sense of worthiness due to subconscious limiting beliefs formed during our early years.

One way to discover worthiness as an issue is to notice areas in your life where you have settled.

Many of my divorced clients have told me they knew when they first married that they had "settled." For some, time was running out to have a baby. Others saw all their friends getting married, and thought it was time for them to do the same, or they felt pressured by relatives to "settle down." Some accepted jobs that were not satisfying or spent time with friends who did not reciprocate the care they gave.

Again, I caution to be kind and gentle towards yourself as "settling" choices are reviewed, for building or re-building self-esteem is a process. Many of our perceived deficiencies come from a lack of adequate nurturing during the critical first few years of life. Let go of harsh judgments and know that we do have the power now to change that wiring and not be a victim of the past.

In moving beyond illness, claiming your worthiness to live can impact your health. I recommend clients take these actions:

1. Ask yourself: What would my life look like if I knew I were worthy? Ponder this question for several days and jot down your answers in a journal.

2. Create a vision board of that ideal life, pasting pictures that elevate your emotions to the highest state of feeling as good as possible.

3. Be sure to post a happy picture of yourself on that board, so you see yourself in the vision.

4. Most importantly, put the words I AM WORTHY on that board in capital letters. You need to start training your brain to know it is worthy of your dreams. Look at the vision board four to seven minutes a day, until you get into the feel-good emotion of what you want to manifest.

5. Start tracking daily evidence of new manifestations of worthiness appearing, and express gratitude for the shifts in consciousness. Gratitude journals are a great way to keep emotions elevated to create a new mindset for living.

"If your beliefs are limitless and ever-evolving then your life will be too." —Oprah Winfrey

---

STAYING STRONG

Overcoming fear of recurrence

Believing in the new *mindset for living* requires constant vigilance, particularly within the medical community. Once you have had cancer, normal health visits no longer feel routine for many with whom I have spoken.

Fear of recurrence impacts up to 96 percent of cancer survivors. —Psycho-Oncology Journal, 2013

Unfortunately, just because a cancerous tumor has been removed, does not mean the case is closed. Rather, it often attracts heightened attention by medical professionals who must protect themselves based on their training. Sometimes that means additional tests and procedures will be ordered.

As the psyche continues to adapt to life post cancer, healing can also feel more like the emotional roller coaster one endures through grief. There are good days and bad, and just when you feel on solid footing again, new doubts creep in.

It takes great courage and stamina to assess information, and continually go within and to additional experts for perspective.

Fortunately, there are tools to help calm the mind, as described later in this section.

Deepening Self-Love and Trust

In what was to be a routine yearly mammogram shortly after the two-year anniversary of my lumpectomy, I was waiting a few hours longer than expected outside the x-ray room for results. These lengthy waits are never a good sign. Instead, I was asked to repeat the mammogram, as they saw something "suspicious" on my left breast, which was *not* the one that had a previous tumor removed.

Hours later I met with my breast surgeon who disclosed that this latest mammogram showed "a concentration of calcium deposits in a small area" of my left breast.

My right breast, which had the lumpectomy two years earlier, was completely clear. I felt that should have been a huge celebration given that my surgeon said most recurrence happens within the first two years. I'd done no radiation or drugs, and my breast was clear.

My surgeon confirmed that the left breast particles were not related to the former tumor in my right breast. I left the visit with only confusion.

The Decision Looming Before Me… *Again*

"The truth of the matter is that the solutions to all of our problems and challenges are found in silent communion with God." —Craig Bullock, The Assisi Institute."

Healthcare professionals almost scared me into a quick decision to get that biopsy after my annual mammogram, two years after first being diagnosed with early-stage breast cancer.

In a moment of panic, I booked the appointment for three days later, as offered. Then, 24 hours after that, the choice did not feel right. I had been too rushed. I was scared, but I needed to center within versus try to bypass the fear I was feeling by engaging in a procedure I was unsure was in my best interest at this point.

I called my naturopathic doctor, Dr. George Savastio, who suggested perhaps that I take time to go within, like I did more than two years earlier. At that time, I walked the beach for three weeks solo, seeking inner counsel and comfort.

A biopsy is not just a simple procedure, as is sometimes presented. Rather, it can feel invasive to have a needle inserted into the body. I forgot that part from my previous biopsy— although my breast surgeon assured me biopsies are done differently now, sitting down versus lying on an examine table with your breast hanging uncomfortably over one side as an ultrasound machine is read to locate the area to biopsy.

Still, there is another part to the procedure that feels invasive on a long-term basis. When a biopsy is performed, a tiny metal marker is inserted in the breast for life. That marker does not set off metal detectors in airports, but is recognized worldwide as a locating device for a potential cancer.

Even though this procedure is described in a routine, methodical way, until that visit, I had forgotten that I already had such a device in my right breast.

I hung up the phone from speaking with Dr. Savastio and wrote to my breast surgeon, asking her to clarify where the particles had been found and what size. She wrote back, assuring me these were tiny and "VERY" (the capital letters were hers) different from the tumor found on my other breast.

Relieved, I decided to take more time to ask my body and God what to do, not base my choice on a quick fear-based assessment. The surgeon told me I did not need to rush. I could wait a month, but probably not four months.

Then, I had to do the hardest part of this healing journey: I had to get raw, and feel my fright. **Spiritual leader Deepak Chopra**

says it takes six months after a diagnosis to get grounded again. I didn't have a diagnosis this time, just a recommendation to get a biopsy that could give me a diagnosis. Yet, a diagnosis does not uncover the causes of the imbalance of the body. Rather, biopsies only remove the evidence of the imbalance.

I needed to first see if I could bring my body back into balance rather than rely on the technical advances of mammography and biopsies to make decisions. Part of me felt sure of engaging in an alternative healing path, but another part wondered if I was courting death. Fear stepped in and up.

For the first time ever, I saw my own funeral with my kids at Crane Beach in Ipswich, Massachusetts, tossing my ashes into the sea. That beach has long been my "heaven on earth," the place I walked for miles finding a deeper connection to God. In the puffy clouds above, my soul was lurking briefly, assuring my children that I was happy and experiencing great love and beauty. *"Go forward in life with joy," I tell them, hoping they know this is my greatest wish for them: "Let go, let love continue to expand in your lives. Keep choosing love over fear. Make time for silence so you can hear your own voice and God's guidance. It's always there, just as I will be there for you in a new way."*

I sobbed tears of release, before gaining this insight: **I had no control over outcomes, only in how I live the moments before me.**

After a week of rebellion, eating and drinking whatever I wanted, a wiser part of me urged me to rest and return to a state of love versus fear from the traumatic visit to the doctor.

The trauma is not necessarily from the feedback from the mammogram—although it is scary when medical professionals see anything. The angst begins with the whole scene of waiting in a room with a TV blaring instead of hearing soft music or a healing meditation tape of hope and possibility.

To me, the long wait felt like all the patients were lined up to see if our number would be called. I kept wondering as we each sat alone in silence: *Would any of us be one of the eight women diagnosed with breast cancer? Who will be the lucky ones, told they could go home? Who will be asked to stay, like me, for repeat photographs of their breasts? Why aren't there any nurturing, supportive health professionals teaching patients about the power of their minds to heal, or to calm our bodies?*

Lingering over my choices, a new anger at the conventional medical community emerged for the manner in which information is presented. The words doctors tell us have a major impact on our health and wiring our brain for negative or positive outcomes, as shown in several studies noted in Dr. Joe Dispenza's book, *You Are the Placebo: Making the Mind Matter.*

Why do we train doctors how to diagnose, but not how to deliver the diagnosis? I thought incredulously. *Where is the truth here? Do the doctors know more than we do when we quiet our minds and listen within? How can we learn to better trust ourselves and collaborate with doctors versus hand the power over to them?*

My logical mind kept wondering if indeed the advanced technology of mammograms was a blessing or a curse. It is easy to say mammograms save lives. Statistics show they do. Yet, they steal lives, too—when we lose all innocence about our carefree lives and become instead hypervigilant about our health.

Sadly, many are misdiagnosed with cancers they do not have, as reported in the past in the *New York Times* and other newspapers, and end up with treatments that hurt other parts of their bodies. For example, we all have cancer cells in our bodies. Some disappear on their own. Or "crystals" like mine may appear on one mammogram, and then never again show up.

Pondering what to do regarding the biopsy, I took time off to play, totally detaching from all "thinking." I spent three gorgeous summer days bike riding and walking in nature, dining at sidewalk cafes, laughing and "getting giddy," as my friends would describe.

Then, I returned to a Tong Ren healing circle (as described earlier), immersed in the hope and optimism of the group who supported my vision for perfect health. I also returned to my healthy diet, forgiving myself for digressing in a moment of panic about my health.

A few days later my psyche took another spiral. I learned one of the breast cancer survivors I had met two years earlier in a healing circle had died. It was the first loss I had experienced within my healing community.

When first diagnosed, like me, she was offered "the gold plan" of radiation and Tamoxifen. Her breast cancer later spread to her lung, and then she got a brain tumor. She told me after we first met that she wished she never did the radiation, and aligned instead with her mind's ability to help heal her body.

Another of my breast cancer friends also took "the gold plan" a step further and did chemotherapy after her early-stage breast cancer diagnosis eight years prior. Being a nurse, she was a strong advocate of using all medical intervention possible. Then she reached the more critical Stage-IV three years after that. The cancer had spread to her liver, and she later died. She told me she wished she had made lifestyle changes years earlier instead of relying on drugs.

My friend's death hit me harder than expected, bringing me to some raw places of my soul that I thought I had healed. Initially, there were the "life-in-review" moments: *Did I do enough to help or show I care?*

Then, there was the survivor guilt. *How come cancer took her life yet I am still alive?*

Moving through day three of grief, I realized I would never see my friend again. The finality of her passing flooded me with emotions, from sadness over the loss, to joy at remembering fun moments together.

Her death also reminded me of my own mortality, triggering me back to that stressful day when I first received the diagnosis. All sorts of new doubts began creeping in: *Will my wellness routine work? Have I done enough to keep my body cancer-free?*

Upon first getting diagnosed with cancer, I took life by the reins and chose to live as fully and healthily as possible. Yet, I have not always been able to stay on track, even though I probably live healthier than 90 percent of the population. *Will that 10 percent of imperfection impact my longevity?* I wondered.

After wallowing in sorrow, fear, and low vibration energies for a few days, I reminded myself that grief for the loss of a friend was healthy. I believe in staying positive, knowing that our thoughts and feelings create our lives.

I also know from decades of coaching others that we do not jump through grief or other negative emotions, particularly those hardwired into us from earlier conditioning, to higher levels of gratitude and joy in an instant. We must feel our negative emotions in order to release them.

Instead of distracting myself from feeling my feelings by immersing in work or other activities, I let the hurt and sadness flow through me, and I honestly articulated what I was feeling. Some people could not handle the less-than-positive side of me and disappeared. Other friends were lovingly supportive and non-judgmental.

I moved slowly and pampered myself as I released those heavier emotions. At the end of the day, I swam for an hour, taking breaks to sit by the edge of the pool and just float in silence. The rippling water from the movement of my body, as I gently swayed my legs in front, gave me a sense of being hugged and rocked like a baby.

I returned home from the pool and meditated for an hour, before drifting off into one of the best night's sleep in a long while.

The next morning when I got up and walked, I felt at peace, grateful for a new day, and expanded and re-committed to my life purpose.

When we take the time to feel our negative emotions as they occur, and release them, we open to the higher feel-good energies like compassion, joy, and love.

What better gift to give those who pass on than a deepening of our own love so we can better serve those who are alive?

What If the Doctor is Wrong?

The loneliness of the cancer-healing journey has sometimes been magnified by not knowing which healthcare professionals to trust to truly care for me. Sometimes, I have felt in a maze of sterile, fast-paced, profit-centered businesses versus the loving hands of a compassionate physician assisting me to stay healthy.

I remember the day my oncologist disapproved of my choice to decline radiation. She first tried scaring me with thoughts the cancer could metastasize. Then, while trying my best to stand firm in my decision to begin first by trying to heal through diet and self-care, she told me she could not support my path. In fact, she said that "new age diet stuff" has nothing to do with cancer.

Doctors, to protect themselves I am told, have to offer the pharmaceutical-based "gold plan." Interestingly, none are held accountable when it does not work.

Yet, I know many survivors who are thriving after radiation decades later.

So how does one know who to trust?

Going the alternative route offers no guarantees or clear-cut answers either. Just as there is money to be made with pharmaceuticals—and cancer *is* big business—there is money to be made with supplements that naturopathic doctors frequently prescribe and sell at a mark-up as well.

Supplements are helpful at the beginning of diagnosis to help bring the body more rapidly back into balance until proper nutrition is established. Long-term, however, many healers I spoke with believe it is best to take in nutrients from whole, unprocessed foods.

The nurturing care I received from my initial naturopathic doctor was superb. His empathy and compassion, along with his healing wisdom in ancient modalities, contributed greatly to my health. Yet, I had an experience with another naturopath who charged me $795 for an office visit plus supplements two weeks before my biopsy.

"Two weeks of supplements can alter a biopsy result?" I asked incredulously. He affirmed that yes, indeed, being aggressive with the supplements he was suggesting could affect the results of whether my suspicious speck was cancerous or not. I later polled a few other naturopaths I respect who thought it was unlikely supplements could make an impact in that short period of time.

Worse, this naturopath had the wrong patient's chart in front of him when he met me, and began our appointment by sending me into post-traumatic stress, which took days from which to recover.

"Given that you have cancer, would you still do the same route today that you have done in the past?" he asked.

Shocked, thinking he was reading from my recent mammogram report, I sat there stunned. He was telling me I had cancer after being cancer-free for nearly three years.

"What do you mean by that, that I have cancer?" I asked, wondering what he saw in the lab report in front of him that I had not been told about.

He looked up, and then apologized. He immediately summoned an office staff member to his office, asking that my correct chart of information be brought in.

Hearing the words '*You have cancer*' is a traumatic event. There was nothing he could do in that moment to rewind the stress he caused. I was so shaken I could barely think.

After weeks of preparing his lengthy forms for my records to be sent to him, along with my latest mammogram results, he had not even spent time reviewing my information beforehand. He said he could not possibly invest that time upfront, but at the next visit we could look more thoroughly at my medical history.

For the cost of an office visit—which I had to pay out-of-pocket, as insurance did not cover his care—to not have a doctor know one thing about me as a new patient when I sat in front him was shocking.

Later over lunch with a friend, the anger welled up inside of me, and I called the office demanding a total refund for the visit and supplements. I was first told I could return the supplements and be credited, but had to pay for the visit. I could speak with the doctor directly if I wanted. I explained that unless he refunded the doctor fee, too, I would pursue other action.

I explained to the office manager who returned my call that the doctor never reviewed my file and he caused great anxiety by saying I had cancer when my mammogram showed me to be cancer-free. She said he corrected himself later but I reiterated that did not undo the jolting scare. His lack of remorse for sending me into shock was even more appalling. Later, I got a call offering to give me a full refund, which was honored.

Sometimes, in the vulnerability that comes with having been a cancer patient, I have felt preyed upon—to be made money from in a fear-based medical system—instead of the empowered woman I have become who would very much like to be acknowledged.

It takes enormous strength to be in a medical setting and keep listening within for guidance amidst others in authority positions. Sadly, just because health professionals have initialed credentials next to their names, does not mean they can be trusted.

So which doctor do you trust? I must continue to go within and access the wisdom of my body through quiet. Then, I must align with healthcare professionals who support my own wisdom along with their expertise.

"Each patient carries his own doctor inside him. They come to us not knowing that truth. We are at our best when we give the doctor who resides within each patient a chance to go to work."—Dr. Albert Schweitzer

WHEN IS ENOUGH, ENOUGH?

Here we go again into what feels like medical madness.

When the "specks" did not disappear after six months of trying to balance my body, the new radiologist in Arizona looked me directly in the eyes and firmly said, "You need to have a biopsy." The new naturopathic doctor, who also tried selling me hundreds of dollars of supplements, had concurred without ever having seen my mammogram, by just reading the recommendation of the radiologist. I am told naturopaths do not read mammograms, anyway.

So. I had the biopsy and did other healing modalities to help me release any emotional toxins lingering in my body (using the energy healers cited in earlier chapters).

The biopsy showed my specks to be cancer-free, but over the long-term there is a 20 percent chance cancer could appear on the spot to the left of where the specs were tested. My breast surgeon suggested, to be safe, that I have an MRI-led surgery procedure to remove it.

Seriously? There was no suspicion of this area in the mammogram or ultrasound performed three weeks earlier. Yet now there are flipped statistics. On the examining table, they said there is an 80 percent chance the biopsy would show my specks were benign, meaning only a 20 percent chance they would be cancerous.

Damn it. Can't I just relish in the joy of being told there is 'no cancer' in my left breast, after finally acquiescing to a biopsy? Now I have both breasts showing no cancer. There has been no recurrence, a huge cause of celebration!

Now, instead of focusing on the 80 percent chance this "new doubt" (as I have called it instead of the scary technical term the message used) is nothing to be concerned about, the doctor is targeting the 20 percent chance it "could" develop into cancer. Umm, is there something not right? I am starting to feel like I am at a Blackjack table trying to beat the odds, even though they are greatly in my favor. With an 80 percent chance of nothing wrong again, just like my specks proved to be, I am still being recommended for another invasive surgical procedure. Opening the breast again feels risky.

I am unsure now if my health is really at stake, or if I am just another potential money-making procedure, for by this point in my near three years journey of healing cancer, I do know that cancer is big business. Not every doctor—whether conventional or alternative—can be trusted. I will always have to look out (or better yet, "within") for myself and align with God for answers.

Is all this looking for "what's wrong?" through the latest advances in diagnostic equipment really a positive step forward in health? Could patients heal faster by focusing on what is right and good?

My brain was not even given one minute to absorb my good news of being cancer-free, which to me was a huge victory and validation of my healing path working.

I wanted to celebrate all the hard inner work I did to remove emotional toxins that may have contributed to any imbalance in my body. Instead, the joy was thwarted briefly by being left with a second part of my good news message that included "a hook of doubt" as I will remember the voicemail. The next day, I intentionally chose to ignore the second part of the message and re-center in connecting with my body's innate ability to stay healthy.

Hence, I did not call the surgeon back right away. Instead, I went out and played, calling friends, took long gratitude walks in nature, and toasted my good news.

Six days later, on a Sunday night after a relaxing, peaceful weekend appreciating the health of my body, the surgeon left another message, suggesting I make an appointment to discuss the possibility of another operation.

Angry that the peace and calm I was again enjoying was tainted by this call on a Sunday night no less, I sobbed into my pillow. Tossing and turning all night, I kept asking myself: *Do I want to keep getting tested, poked at, and looking to see what may go wrong in future years? What is the value of living life now, in the moment, embracing my good health and the peaceful, loving life style, which I have created?*

After hours of reviewing options, I made this decision upon awaking from a restless night: I called my surgeon back on her cell phone from which she left her message instead of her business line where she asked me to call to set up an appointment. I calmly left the message on Monday morning, March 23: *"Dr......., This is Gail Jones. I wanted to confirm that I got both of your messages, the one when the biopsy report came in, and the Sunday call last night. You said there was no urgency to doing the next procedure. I have decided that I would like to keep my body in a state of peace and calm. You had already scheduled a follow-up mammogram prior to the biopsy for August. I would like to review my information then (five months from now) and consider an MRI (which is less harmful to the body, my research shows) then instead of that mammogram.*

In choosing to just "be" a while, and integrate the good feelings of health in my body, I am also deciding to claim emotionally that I am enough, have done enough, and do not have to keep reaching, striving for perfection. A doctor later validated my choice, saying I made a smart decision: opening the breast for such low odds is risky.

Living every waking moment trying to control the outcome of health is not "living."

Ammunition Against the Fear

Reducing fight-or-flight with Bill Harris' Holosync®

Do everything to calm the lymphatic system.

Staying calm, and out of the fight-or-flight high adrenaline emotions that sometimes accompany the cancer healing journey, takes great tenacity at times.

Despite my best efforts to recreate life beyond cancer from a new foundation of self-love and worthiness, I still had some fearful moments like millions of others diagnosed.

I occasionally face heightened states of stress from fear of recurrence. To deal with my anxiety and conduct research for this book, I began practicing Holosync brain wave technology from Centerpointe Research Institute for six months initially and later returned to it periodically.

Childhood trauma also can make one's threshold for stress lower, sending one into fight-or-flight states more easily, according to Bill Harris, founder of Centerpointe and creator of Holosync. Learning to slow down has been key to healing as well as the messages and practices I teach as a transformational coach and wellness pioneer.

"The more trauma, the lower your threshold—and the more often you'll be triggered by circumstances and life events that might not bother someone with a higher threshold," Harris claims.

Difficult emotions—anger, fear, depression, confusion, addictions, overeating, and many others—are really just attempts to cope with being pushed over your personal threshold for what you can handle, according to Harris.

The solution, he says, is to raise your threshold higher by activating your parasympathetic nervous system to keep your sympathetic nervous system from sending you into fight-or-flight mode.

When practiced regularly for an hour a day for a minimum of four to six months, Holosync can help you become calmer, have more energy and think more clearly by inducing "the relaxation response" within the body more often, he maintains.

Some results he noticed are that when people are less stressed, they become kinder, more compassionate, and happier with a mind that works better.

"Eventually you get to the point that what used to bother you feels like it happened to someone else; you can remember it and learn from it, but will not be so charged," Harris asserts. "The prefrontal cortex learns from experience and you don't need to release over and over again the 'echo' of traumatic experience."

For cancer patients, strengthening the pre-frontal cortex in the brain is especially important.

"When somebody has cancer, they go into fight-or-flight, which makes a lot of cortisol that interferes with the immune system," Harris says. "Holosync helps calm the lymphatic system that puts a person in fight-or-flight, with users eventually observing circumstances more dispassionately."

"The more calm you can be, the more you can fight off the cancer," he stresses. "You don't need to create more cortisol."

Living in fight-or-flight from a poor lymphatic system also often contributes to lack of will power, Harris claims. More specifically, an overactive lymphatic system creates more dopamine which causes people to do things without looking at the consequences— such as eating things not good for them, spending money they don't have, saying things in anger, skipping exercise, engaging with social media instead of working on their business, and not making plans and sticking with them.

"You have to learn not to be driven by dopamine—and instead focus on long range and delayed gratification and being steadfast," Harris says, citing the 2009 Stanford *Zero to Three* study of preschoolers.

That study shows those who would not touch candy and wait (and get a greater reward of more candy later for waiting, which was only 15 percent of those tested) had better grades, better health, higher SAT scores, lower body mass, and could set goals and achieve them. The brain scans of those who could wait also showed they had strong pre-frontal cortexes and a calm lymphatic system. Those who couldn't wait got into more trouble.

A strong pre-frontal cortex also reduces the amount of fearful thoughts that people get sucked into, and helps them become more aware to make better choices that increase happiness, and be more loving, he says.

When asked how his Holosync technology differs from other meditative practices from the new field of neuroscience that have been tracking significant relaxation shifts in users, he says many of those techniques are based on changing the mindset of a person. Holosync, on the other hand, actually changes the brain waves, he claims.

MY RESULTS of Practicing Level One—The Holosync Prologue for six months:

First, I had to buy a good headset, which must be worn to experience the balancing of the left and right sides of the brain.

Second, the company suggests it is best to do the meditation the same time every day, either morning or evening, to make it a routine. I found the morning time often helped me set the day off on a more optimistic, centered tone. When I did the meditation in the evening, I was able to sleep better. I mixed it up, spending a few weeks listening to Holosync in the morning, and then shifting for the next couple of weeks to meditating in the evening.

Initially, while practicing for one hour a day, I had many raw moments of release of emotions, particularly grief over the past. Harris recommended that I keep trying to step aside and observe the circumstances, become curious and not resist the emerging feelings. Resisting activates fight-or-flight, he said. Eventually, knee-jerk feelings lessen, although the more trauma one has experienced, the more difficult it can be to step back and allow yourself to feel your stuckness, he noted.

Observations of changes after one week (began mid-June 2015): I was becoming softer, moving more slowly, making clearer choices, continuing to be the "witness" of my life versus "reactor," who in the past sometimes responded too quickly to emotions.

The following weeks, I experienced more time walking through "dark nights of the soul." It seemed many repressed emotions from being an unmothered daughter and how alone and scared I truly felt came up. Living in WITNESS MODE I saw my defenses and perfectionist standards more clearly, as I continued to lighten up and pace myself.

Over the longer term, I consistently became calmer. Some days I reached pure levels of bliss, increasingly experiencing greater joy.

Specifics of my ongoing progress include:

- Driving in strange places feeling calmer, like when visiting my son for Parents' Weekend at his college in upstate New York, traveling on highways I've never been on to see him.

- Sleeping better through the night, thinking less about recurrence and more about expressing my life purpose.

- Becoming more disciplined—and with greater clarity, taking inspired actions.

- Stopping more often to discern if an opportunity is the right move for me.

- Feeling more centered in myself, yet also more strategic (like bringing someone with me to health appointments for support, asking for help when needed, listening more and talking less).

- Gaining more clarity on the types of relationships I want (consistent, grounded, happy people who can empathize and reciprocate). More letting go of my past pattern of putting others' needs before my own.

- Sensing an UPGRADE to my life occurring as I connect with higher quality people and opportunities.

- Experiencing more pleasant, sometimes even conciliatory dreams, of people from the past who may have hurt me.

At times, I used the tool to self-soothe versus cling to others for support. I became kinder to others and myself and less judgmental.

I also started a gratitude practice after listening to the meditations, jotting down each day five things that I appreciate about my life or the people in it.

As I continued beyond the six-month trial, I increasingly felt more rested and needed less sleep, and was better able to focus after using Holosync. Due to the one-hour daily time commitment, and my interest in exploring other healing tools as research for this book, I stopped using Holosync for several months.

I noticed when I started using it again I felt happier, and more detached from stressful situations, like living in the unknown through the process of reinvention. Hence, I've incorporated the meditation back into my life on a near daily basis.

No matter what anyone tells me about my medical reasons for getting cancer, I continue to believe my fight-or-flight mode of operating from early childhood conditioning (and literally fleeing from my mom) wore my body down.

I had to stop to rest and heal. I made two pit stops—downsizing to Newburyport, Massachusetts, to come alive in new ways and choose love for myself, then later moving to Scottsdale, Arizona, for the peace of simple outdoor living, ease of getting around, and happy people in sunshine during the winter months.

For more information about Holosync:
Centerpointe Research Institute, Beaverton, OR
www.centerpointe.com

REDUCING FEAR BY RESTORING SURVIVOR'S HOPE – DR. SHANI FOX

"Cancer demands the most you can give; so much strength and persistence. That can be exhausting at the time, but that very same strength, persistence, and the wisdom you gather in the process can be leveraged to create a life that really reflects the best of you. My job is to restore survivors' hope and help them move beyond fear to reclaim their lives on their terms, not cancer's terms." —Dr. Shani Fox, www.drshanifox.com, whose practice is 100 percent focused on cancer survivors.

There is a nagging secret many survivors live with that even those closest to them often cannot understand: cancer may go away, but not the scary thought that it could return at any time no matter what we do as survivors to stay healthy.

Sadly, up to 96 percent of the 14 million cancer survivors in the U.S. today live with persistent fear of recurrence according to research noted in the 2013 edition of *Psycho-Oncology Journal.*

"We need to take the fear statistics seriously," says Dr. Shani Fox, a leading holistic physician, life mastery coach, and expert in cancer survivorship. "Fear is ruining a lot of lives. There are people who dread getting out of bed in the morning, and can't wait to get back into bed so they don't have to face the fear. Others have panic attacks. Fear is very widespread, even among survivors who are healthy and have low chance of recurrence, as I've seen in my practice."

To address this issue, Dr. Fox created The Cancer Survivor's Fear First Aid Kit™. She says her product is especially helpful in moving survivors from the fight-or-flight mode of high anxiety that accompanies fear of cancer recurrence to the more nurturing "rest and digest" state, where they can embrace the joy of living today.

The Kit is a three-part offering that includes a 28-page book detailing her simple, five-step method for quickly reducing fear of cancer recurrence, a companion workbook to help survivors learn the method quickly and track their progress, and a CD with guided meditation audio tracks to help survivors integrate the book's lessons and succeed in overcoming their fears.

To learn more, check out:
drshanifox.com/the-cancer-survivors-fear-first-aid-kit/

"Reducing stress is an essential part of every cancer survivor's prevention program," Dr. Fox notes. "This Kit addresses a particularly common and stubborn form of stress among survivors: fear of recurrence."

Helping survivors address other emotional issues of recreating their lives after cancer is another gap she fulfills beyond treatment offered by conventional Western medicine.

"Western medicine is all about the body," she says. "Yet, a very large dimension of the survivor's experience is at the level of the emotions. We ignore or undertreat that at our peril."

The mainstays of Western medicine, surgery and pharmaceuticals, aren't widely applicable in survivorship, she maintains. "What ails cancer survivors doesn't resolve with medication," Dr. Fox asserts. "People are simply experiencing normal physical and emotional responses to life-changing circumstances. And yet, it can be very hard to move through and beyond these responses—especially the anxiety and fear—to feeling serene and joyful without some support."

Dr. Fox's approach is to help her clients master the body's normal fear response, deciding how much attention they allocate to it.

"If we stay in panic, it's because we're conditioned to run away from fear," Dr. Fox explains. "As long as we continue to see fear as bad, we're locked into struggle with it. We'll exhaust ourselves continually running from it. Ultimately, we need to be willing to turn around and face the fear: find out what it's doing there, find out what it wants to tell us."

She says this inner journey is best not done alone, as persistent fear is typically there for a reason that may require outside perspective to discern. Trying to pretend the fear is not there is not helpful, either.

"People are always telling survivors to think positive," she shares. "That's not great advice for a cancer survivor, and survivors know it. It's not possible nor is it realistic to be positive all the time. Life isn't positive all the time. It's not about 100 percent positivity; it's about 100 percent authenticity."

Even though cancer can be scary and she in no way undermines the hard challenges of it, she encourages survivors to look for the blessings in the experience, the beneficial parts that may have moved their lives forward in some way. She believes survivors can surpass "a new normal" to attain "a new extraordinary."

"Life is in the moments," she says. "Life is in the days. I train my survivors to remember that life is right now. Is right now the way I want it, or do I want something different?"

Helping survivors discover their authentic selves is Dr. Fox's passion and supports the results her clients have achieved in renewing their health. Many have returned to long-lost dreams like becoming an artist or discovered new callings like saving a rare wildlife species, living more happily after cancer than before. Her concluding words are even more assuring:

"Part of shifting from a fear-driven life to a love-driven life is being willing to believe in your own magnificence. That's a belief I help people cultivate: you contain magnificence. It's very difficult to see sometimes, particularly after an experience like cancer, when your body and any number of things may have changed in ways you don't recognize. And yet, your core magnificence is absolutely still there. That's a part of you that cancer does not touch."

MOVING FORWARD TO THE NEW LIFE

"As a spiritual aspirant, when you have a serious illness you realize that it is time to do some significant work on yourself. You understand that it is important to let go as deeply as you can because you may not have much time left. Your predicament helps you to appreciate the life you have and do the real work to raise yourself spiritually. You let go, with deep love and compassion for your humanness, with the understanding that this may or may not heal the cancer, but more importantly, it heals your entire being."

—Michael A. Singer, author of *The Untethered Soul* and *The Surrender Experiment*

Mourning life as I knew it

For all the ways my life has improved as I recreated myself post cancer, there are two losses that I continually wrestle with: loss of freedom and loss of control.

I can no longer live my life in whatever way I want without considering there could be life or death consequences. Having that thought hang over my head daily is restrictive. Finding the balance between making conscious choices and being a perfectionist is a tough act.

Some new choices are easier than others.

Increasing my exercise to at least 30 minutes of aerobic activity five days a week is fun and often rejuvenating—especially if I am engaged in outdoor fitness. Yet, adhering to new dietary restrictions continues to be a challenge. I am not the purist I intended to be as noted in previous chapters. That loss of freedom of eating and drinking whatever I want sometimes seems like a small price to pay for an extended life. Yet, how I want to live in joy and celebration sometimes puts me in conflict of whether to indulge or not in a great piece of dark chocolate or glass of red wine. My higher conscience does not always win—making me angry at myself for not being as self-disciplined as intended.

Another cancer survivor I spoke with says to this day she still beats herself up for having an ice cream cone a few years back.

The other loss, the perception that I have or had control over my life, got tossed with the cancer diagnosis. No longer was I humming along or pushing forward, which was more my style. In fact, I probably never felt so out of control in my life as during those scary days waiting for the pathology reports, knowing my fate was in God's hands, the ultimate surrender.

Did I do enough healing beforehand? Did I truly forgive everyone I could, including myself? Did I pray hard enough, say enough affirmations of perfect health, and visualize enough about my ideal health? Eventually, I came to understand that I had to surrender all those thoughts to truly live in the moment.

Dr. Jennifer Irwin, a professor, researcher on behavioral change, spouse, mother, grandparent, a daughter of two cancer survivors, and a cancer survivor herself, says the emotional impact of a cancer diagnosis is profound and that doctors rarely offer ways to deal with hearing the life-altering news. Patients can feel horrifically betrayed by their body and "every single thing in your life is different from that point on," she observed. "You now have changes in your life—maybe you just have to feel what you are going through."

Cancer is a gift, wrapped in barbed wire.
—Lance Armstrong

The added burden is figuring out how to integrate the role of survivor with other roles in life. "There is no manual for how to be a survivor," Dr. Irwin notes. "There is not a right way to do survivorship. It's about finding what sits most comfortably in your gut, your way." For her, she found being a survivor easier than being the caretaker for two survivors. Yet, loss of control for someone who had a life and retirement well-planned was most challenging.

"Your sense of control shifts as that day of diagnosis, everything about your schedule changes. You have to roll with everything being different. Your perspectives shift and your way of operating in the world change. There can be an opening of your world or a terror of the world, which can depend on what day you're in."

Dr. Irwin suggests survivors explore loss of control by asking:

- Where do you find your life has been disrupted?
- What time is not your own?
- Where do you feel you have no choice?

Other losses include:

- Privacy and boundaries: "You can't turn your ringer off; sometimes you need to wait to hear about an appointment."
- Expectations in relationships: The experience is hard to explain to other people.
- Cancer is not something you choose to have, yet you are forced to deal with all the "new normal."
- Loss of control over how this impacts those around you, particularly when survivors may need or choose to put themselves first to heal. Dr. Irwin recalls saying to her husband: "I need to be selfish here and I will need to lean on you. You have to get support for what you are going through around this somewhere else."

Finding ways to "park resentment" and forgive yourself is important. "You did not do this to yourself. There is no cure for all the cancers in the world."

"Some days are great because I forget I once had cancer. And some days are great I because I remember I had cancer... There is not a right or wrong way to do it—and I don't know anyone who has done it without some hiccups."
—Dr. Jennifer Irwin

Inspiration from a Long-Term Survivor

Rose Russo

Meeting like-minded others who made similar lifestyle choices helped me stay the course of trusting in my body's innate ability to heal. Rose Russo is one of those inspiring women who became both a friend and colleague. Founder of Pathways—Life as Art, Rose is a visual artist, graphic designer, Anusara yoga instructor, energy healer practitioner, and two-time cancer survivor.

She generously offers a monthly, by-donation-only, "Yoga Hope for Cancer Patients, an Exploration in Self-healing and Mindfulness" at the Yoga center where she teaches in Newburyport, Massachusetts.

Today, Rose is thriving in health 23 years after her cancer diagnosis, without using any drugs, radiation, or chemotherapy—bold choices she made after watching her father die years earlier from colon cancer.

She attributes her healing success to having a belief system in place that honored the wisdom of her body and gave her the courage to buck medical authority.

"I listened to my body the whole time," she shares. "I have a sensitive system with a strong reaction to modern medicine and I didn't want to put my body through what I saw my father endure with his colon cancer treatments. What conventional doctors were doing wasn't healing in the case of my father. They were managing the effects of the cancer's growth and slow decay of his body. Those observations led me to look and say that I am not going to do that. There must be a better way."

Rose notes she was fortunate that her breast cancer was diagnosed at an early stage, which gave her more options for healing. Still, her path to wellness involved enormous amounts of stamina and an inner soul search that transformed her life to the point where she now calls cancer "a blessing."

"Cancer changed my life," she states. "It needed to be changed. I learned so much from going through this experience and I teach from the place of blessing and not from a place of fear."

Prior to her diagnoses, she lived a workaholic lifestyle, with too much time spent getting tasks done, sitting in front of the computer learning new technical skills and not enough time in nature, movement, silence, or conscious eating or being.

"After the diagnosis, I went through the 'Oh My God, my body failed me' place," Rose says. "It felt like a loss of innocence. I could not go about my day without being conscious of what I was doing to my body. You cannot abuse it and expect to be okay. And I needed to learn to be more conscious in all the things I was doing."

Walking the beach everyday at sunset and learning yoga at age 49 brought her life back to balance and gave her renewed purpose, as she, too, learned to live from the heart.

First diagnosed in 1994 with invasive, intra-ductal, Stage-I breast cancer at the age of 42, Rose proceeded with a lumpectomy but to the dismay of her doctors she declined the recommended conventional treatment and Tamoxifen often used as an approach to keep cancer from recurring. The doctors could not convince her otherwise, Rose says, urging patients to be sure to ask key questions about long-term consequences upfront before agreeing to any treatment.

"I asked my doctor if she had 100 percent cured, or 50 percent cured or 25 percent success with this treatment, and she said 'No.' So I created a letter stating I would not sue her. She gave me her recommendations, but I chose not to take those options, and asked her to at least do the surgeries/lumpectomies for me. I took 100 percent responsibility for my own healing regimen and health."

Angry that Rose declined Tamoxifen, the doctor insisted Rose speak to a radiologist, which led Rose to probe further for definitive answers. "I asked him a number of questions, 'If I do not do radiation and cancer comes back, what are my options?' He said I'd have all the options available because the tissue wouldn't have been damaged by radiation. I then asked, 'If I were a person who did radiation, and the cancer came back, what would my options be then?' He said I'd have to have a mastectomy because the tissue would have been damaged. I asked if radiation would only stay in the area or if my heart and lungs would also be affected. He said they would be, that they couldn't pin the radiation down to just the breast area."

Rose chose to have a lumpectomy to have the cancerous area removed, without adding any follow-up drugs, radiation, or chemotherapy.

Sadly, her surgeries included not one, but four lumpectomies over a six-month period, as the doctor was unable to get clear margins on the first attempt to remove the cancer. The doctor also took out 23 lymph nodes instead of checking the first three removed to determine if all the cancer had been captured, causing severe scars that were later clear in subsequent surgeries.

Some doctors, Rose explains, believe the fewer lymph nodes that need to be removed to see if the cancer has spread, the better, to keep the lymph system functioning optimally. Luckily, to this day Rose has not experienced any lymphedema—dangerous swelling which frequently occurs when so many lymph nodes have been removed. She credits not having radiation in that area, which allowed the lymph system to find a natural way to drain.

She began by researching vitamins and herbs, including Essiac, a tea which she drank every day. Comprised of four main herbs—Burdock Root, Slippery Elm Inner Bark, Sheep Sorrel, and Indian

Rhubarb Root—the original Essiac formula is believed to have its origins from the native Canadian Ojibway Indians. It is named after Rene Caisse ("Essiac" spelled backwards), a Canadian nurse who pulled together the herbs after witnessing a woman experience healing from breast cancer with no recurrence. Today, Essiac can be found in many health food stores, and prices vary dramatically depending on the brand.

Then, Rose changed her diet, both what and how she ate, slowing down to cook nutritious meals, with a lot more alkaline-based foods like broccoli, less meat (which is like a "sweet" to the body), salmon, and fruits.

Rose also learned Reiki, a Japanese technique for stress reduction and relaxation that is said to promote healing through "the laying on of hands" that enables life force energy to flow through a patient. Through greater introspection, she was able to identify the major stressors in her life.

Then five years later, cancer was again identified on her left breast through a routine mammogram.

"You have many options, to look at this as a victim or to look at this as something you are supposed to learn and share— especially the second diagnosis which hit me harder," Rose says. "I realized I had to go even deeper within and continue to discover new ways to stay healthy."

She also reduced her stress further by transferring all her care and medical records from Boston to a local hospital nearby where she lived. She found two incredible local surgeons, who agreed to treat her with a "free care" option due to her recent loss of income. Then, she paused for two weeks and listened quietly for answers within, before choosing her next steps for healing.

Still adamant about not using drugs, radiation, or chemotherapy, Rose embarked on a mastectomy (on her left breast only) called a "transflap," an older surgery no longer performed today the way it was done then. It involved using Rose's own body—including large rectus and abdominal muscles as a filler versus employing silicone implants, which at the time were having problems with leakages.

"The surgeons understood I was doing my own thing and they were willing to be a support to me," Rose explained. "In fact, the first appointment after surgery, my doctor's nurse cried when she saw how well I was doing. And, to this day, my doctor still says I am her 'star' patient."

Recovering from surgery, she used sound healing, self-applied Reiki, and visualizations focused on walking the beach. These techniques were so helpful to her recovery that she was released from the hospital a day early. Rose also limited the number of people with whom she shared this second diagnosis and surgery to eliminate any negativity feedback.

Her subsequent healing journey from her second bout with breast cancer led Rose to deepen her spiritual practice with inspirational readings every day, committing to staying positive, and surrounding herself with people who could be "life supporting." She also deepened and practiced her feelings of self-love.

"I needed to embrace a kinder view of myself, a more worthy sense of self-love, which was missing," Rose shares, claiming up until her cancer diagnosis, she had been very hard on herself, driven by her ego versus her spirit, to be self-sufficient and make a living.

To stay more connected to spirit she chose to refrain from stresses like listening to the radio, news on TV, or advertisements and opted instead to tune into quieter and calmer, introspective types of music and activities.

Basically, Rose "narrowed her life" with better boundaries for healing by focusing on what she could do to help her body live within what she calls "a toxic world." Good food, less stressors, exercise, meditating outdoors (even in winter), and yoga have led Rose to her healthy new way of life.

Plus, yoga is a sustainable practice, which is important to Rose, along with other self-healing modalities like meditation, crystals, flower essence, and energy healing. She says, "You need to touch the stone of healing every day."

Through yoga, Rose slowly became strong enough after surgery to enjoy her longer walks on the beach.

To this day, 23 years after first diagnosed with cancer, Rose will not turn on her computer on weekends. Instead, she embraces her downtime and teaches Yoga Hope for cancer patients (either currently in treatment or years beyond) one Saturday per month to cancer patients as her way of serving.

"Part of the reason I decided to teach yoga is to help people find and stay healthy. That requires a connection within, to move the body's energy on a regular basis and to find joy in moving. Yoga gave me all of that."

Her work in sharing self-healing concepts helps bridge the gap for many patients, who after completing a medical health regimen or treatment, are at a loss on how to move forward in their lives.

"I have seen more people fall into old habits and have a recurrence of cancer during this time period after treatment because they have not embraced their own self-healing practices which will sustain them for the rest of their life."

Through her two bouts of cancer—and yoga, mindfulness, and energy work with hundreds of patients—Rose offers a few other suggestions for those newly diagnosed:

1. **BREATHE**. First, take a deep breath and allow yourself to be angry, hurt, sad and all the things that go with hearing that diagnosis.

2. **STAY OPEN:** Don't close yourself off to anything... healing comes in many forms.

3. **CENTER IN SELF**: Do not allow others to lay their fears at your feet or "tell you" what to do. Well-meaning family and friends who have not been diagnosed with cancer often out of fear, fear of losing you, or fear of what they would do if they were in your shoes, may tell you what to do. But only you know what it feels like to have this diagnosis. In the end, this is your healing journey to wholeness and health.

4. **ASK YOURSELF TO BE PLACED IN AS MANY PRAYER GROUPS AS POSSIBLE:** The healing power of prayer has been known to change outcomes.

Most importantly, Rose encourages those diagnosed with cancer to reevaluate their entire lives.

"You were meant to be transformed by this experience. Allow yourself to flow to a new way of being," she says. "Your cancer diagnosis might be the best thing that happened in your life."

To learn more about Rose Russo, visit:
www.pathwayslifeasart.com

MY REINVENTION...

Forgiveness continues...

I saw a few butterflies while walking this morning, thinking they were messages from my mother. I had been asking for signs of her help as I wrote the content related to love in this book. Mom had wanted to be a teacher, and now I am being intuitively guided to serve in that role.

On Earth, my mother was the person who caused me the most pain (or at least feelings of terror). Yet, she also initiated me into my most profound healing. I finally had to learn to stand alone, trusting in God or a Higher Power as my source of support.

Butterflies also have symbolized for me joy and freedom to soar. I am truly grateful my mother is soaring somewhere else now, out of a brain-diseased body.

As I continue to embrace compassion for myself, I look back with love for this woman who was given a challenging health condition. She never got to really know her children or grandchildren; her life was a haze. Emotional connection was nearly impossible.

When I became a mother, my number one priority was "being there" for my kids, but I didn't always do that right either. Sometimes I gave too much; other times not enough or the right type of love. Sadly, they also endured the pain of their parents divorcing, something I vowed would never happen. It just wasn't in the final script—even though we started out as family living in the picture-perfect, sweet cape-styled house with white picket fence, on a gorgeous setting of fields and flowers. I hope one day my children forgive me for my mistakes. I was not the perfect mother I dreamed, but I was the best I knew how to be.

It has taken me 58 years to say these words: "Bless you, Mom. I am so sorry, for not loving you in the ways I wanted to, and not receiving the love I suspect you wanted to give."

Forgiveness has been two-fold: I had to forgive myself for holding onto the hurt and shame of my mom and her illness, along with forgiving my mom for not taking care of me in the ways a child needs.

I began the forgiveness process years earlier, but as I became closer to God through my cancer-healing journey, I saw more clearly the divinity in knowing how we are connected.

Had I not had the mother I did, I may not have been able to guide so many others through abandonment issues, and now the prompting to urge others to forgive those who hurt them so their bodies can heal.

CONCLUSION

THE FIVE-YEAR MARK
(AND SUPPORTING DATA)

After all the inner work, to detox the negative emotions and create new beliefs, I achieved a state of health at the five-year mark since my diagnosis that surprised even those who tested me.

I share the results hesitantly, for I know our bodies are constantly changing. Plus, this book is not about statistics. Rather, my intention is to share insights, tools, and resources for learning to *live now* in a higher state of being—to make all our days no matter how many we have, more joyful and meaningful.

What is so exciting, however, is the alternative path I chose is now backed by evidence. Here are the results presented to me by Karla L. Birkholz, M.D., who tested me on January 31, 2017, just shy of five years after my diagnosis:

> *"Gail has been incredibly conscientious about doing her daily meditations and following neuroscience technology, along with many other healing modalities. After being diagnosed with breast cancer in 2012, she declined radiation and Tamoxifen and opted for alternative routes, changing her diet and training her mind to heal her body. Her efforts have paid off for her, personally and medically.*
>
> *We assessed Gail's health status recently. Our symptom questionnaire, with most people scoring over 70, came back at less than 20. My colleague, Chris Holly [BSN Health Coach], used galvanic skin response testing to assess Gail's ability to respond to stress[ors] and [measure her biological coherence and biological aversion] to nearly 2000 virtual stimuli. Most people tested have several hundred items creating a biological aversion. Amazingly, Gail's body measured 25, the lowest*

number of potential, personal stressors my partner has ever measured, in hundreds of tests over the years! Her capacity for managing stress was high and 20 different organ systems measured green, meaning they were functioning well. Most pertinent, her breasts were doing great, measuring healthier than most of her other organs!

She is truly doing the work, and her body appreciates it!"

To sit before a doctor and a nurse, and be validated for the many intuitive and alternative choices I made, was a defining moment in my medical journey—and maybe in my life. I was honored, validated, seen, heard, and respected by those highly skilled and competent. I have indeed created a new *mindset for living*!

24 PRACTICAL TIPS ON PREVENTION

1. Get your cell phone off your chest, particularly if you're sticking it inside your bra while dancing or working out.

2. Say bye-bye to underwire bras (no metal next to your breast).

3. Ditch deodorants that contain aluminum.

4. Know these core beliefs: You are worthy. You are lovable. You are significant. You matter. You are competent. Align yourself with others who share those same values and honor your vibration of goodness and love.

5. Eat healthy—as little sugar, wheat, and dairy as possible. Add fruits and veggies to your diet, and grapefruit in particular for preventing breast cancer. (Check with your doctor because some medications may conflict.)

6. Drink 64 ounces of purified water a day.

7. Use glass, instead of plastic, for storage and cooking.

8. Practice self-love. What does it mean to take care of your needs before extending yourself to another? You can't serve others from emptiness. Fill yourself up with love so you have more to genuinely share.

9. Make real, face-to-face connections. Communicating via social media does not constitute a relationship. "Being there" for someone is sometimes inconvenient and entails more than a text message. Yet, it is this level of richness that truly sustains you in good times or bad. Those with pets also are said to live 10 years longer.

10. Schedule downtime to just "be"—at least 20 minutes a day is as important (if not more so) than all the tasks you are doing.

11. Look beyond high impact exercise and add activities that free your neck (from all the hours hunched over computers or with a cell phone to your ear)—yoga, Tai Chi, and Qi Gong are great. Hiking or walking in nature helps nurture the soul as well as stretch the body.

12. Feel your feelings. You have to release the negative ones to make room for all the joy and abundance that is your natural birthright.

13. Forgive yourself and others who have hurt you. Know also that you can forgive someone without staying in a relationship with him or her. Forgiveness can be the most healing thing you can do for your mind, body, and soul.

14. Find ways to open your heart, and keep it open. Heart-centered living creates joy and the unity consciousness that heals. Being guarded, on the other hand, keeps us feeling alone and separate. Risk vulnerability—it connects us to the humanness of one another.

15. Slow down. Be aware of what your senses are showing you—what you are seeing, hearing, feeling, touching, or tasting. Life is in the now. Race around too much and you lose not only the connection to your self, but to all the abundance and love around you.

16. Your inner life will determine your outer life. Taking time to clean it up or imagine the way of being you want to experience in the world is one of the best investments in yourself and your life you can make.

17. Take vitamins D3 and D12 for breast cancer—and get 20 minutes of natural sun a day.

18. Eliminate worry—these thoughts can make us sick.

19. Meditate daily, preferably when in a theta state (like first thing in the morning); repeat positive affirmations while looking in a mirror. Closing your eyes after a few deep breaths and scanning the body helps you get into theta state.

20. Practice deep breathing from the lower abdomen throughout the day.

21. Create a vision board of your ideal life and focus on it several minutes a day—train your brain to seek new outcomes.

22. Join a support group of like-minded others. Those in mind-body programs can live as much as 2 to 2.5 times longer than those who are not. Other studies show that meeting in small groups at least once a month adds more to happiness than doubling your salary. And, positive energy can change your body's DNA, as the latest research in epigenetics shows.

23. Build circles to have at least four to ten friends.

24. For young girls especially, explore thermograms versus mammograms, to reduced radiation.

THERMOGRAMS

A diagnostic option not readily discussed

Two years after my breast cancer diagnosis, I had my first meeting for an annual exam with a new doctor, who came highly recommended. Going to see a new doctor for the first time can be a vulnerable experience, especially after having had breast cancer. Until my diagnosis, I didn't expect a doctor to find anything wrong. Now, I know I'm not invincible and am indeed mortal!

Staying focused on the positive takes extra vigilance now. Plus, with the mandates to see so many patients per hour, few doctors have the time to give me the loving nurturance that has become a requirement of my health care. Compassion heals, I believe. Studies have shown that the words doctors utter also impact our belief systems and health outcomes. Not all doctors are trained to offer encouraging thoughts of hope and new possibilities.

After my new doctor's very brief exam, I told her I was considering having a thermogram instead of a mammogram. Having declined radiation as a treatment option after my lumpectomy, I was unsure if I wanted to keep receiving radiation from yearly mammograms.

Also, now that I am very small breasted having lost 30-plus pounds through dietary changes, I didn't want my chest painfully squished beneath a machine. Some also believe that type of pressure on breast tissue can also create more cancer cells to form or spread, I have been told.

"I would rather see you forget the mammogram and do nothing than have a thermogram," my new doctor told me.

I left that office totally discouraged, that my doctor had given advice without any research on the imaging tool I wanted to use. Plus, I was in and out in 20 minutes, hardly what I considered a comprehensive exam to determine my state of health. She didn't even order the full laboratory tests that I had been accustomed to getting in the past, including one for diabetes which runs in my family of origin.

I have since had two mammograms, one where I had to wait in the screening room patient area for three hours for results that someone forgot to give me when they had been available hours earlier, I later learned. Instead, the health team ordered an ultrasound as a precaution, even knowing my mammogram they had not yet shown me was clear. I understand now they are required to do so, to protect their own medical liability.

Before that I had a radiologist stand before me telling me that I *must* have a biopsy for a suspicious speck, even though my naturopathic doctor back East was not concerned yet. He had told me to give my body time to balance itself in rest.

Sadly, in fear, I chose the biopsy, where I was placed on an exam table face down, my breast exposed through a large hole, with a roomful of interns watching. The radiologist was on the floor beneath me withdrawing her sample from my breast.

I cried all the way home, feeling like a guinea pig conned into an unnecessary procedure. There was no warmth or care, just a sterile environment with a stoic, cold radiologist leading her team. The biopsy came back cancer-free. I later learned these extra procedures were recommended to protect their own medical liability.

Fast-forward three years. Additional research caused me to question mammography further. For example, the Swiss Medical Board has been especially critical of mammograms in a report claiming 22 percent of women screened will be exposed to false positives and unnecessary treatment.

I have learned from many healthcare professionals that no matter which screening tool is used, early diagnosis is not the same as prevention, which is best achieved through healthful lifestyle changes.

New advances in thermography

Still, I opted this time to schedule my first thermogram after interviewing a few technologists. My mind raced with fear of the unknown. *Will the thermogram show too much information as one naturopathic doctor I know suggests it does? Will it comfort and reassure me more or scare me as the radiologist did who ordered my biopsy a few years back?*

Did all my time spent meditating, going to yoga, hiking, and changing my diet, keep me cancer-free? Did the financial stress of the past five years hurt my body despite my best attempts at calming my mind and body?

Why is something described as a safe and comfortable tool not generally accepted or offered in conventional medicine? How many times do I have to go within and honor my gut versus established, traditional medicine? This was such a lonely journey. I wanted to cry again.

Thankfully, in my research I came across Pam Mathews, who has worked in both traditional radiology since 1970 and now as a technician offering thermograms. She uses a Meditherm camera system, which is registered and licensed by the FDA, an important distinction to note when evaluating who to use to perform a thermogram. Not all technicians use the same type of camera.

Many also are still unaware of the advances with thermograms. In the past, thermograms were thought to have reported too many false positives before M.D. interpreters started reading the images, Mathews explained.

A trained doctor, who then submits the analysis to the patient to give to her chosen physician, reads all Mathews' thermograms.

Now many leading health insurers are recognizing thermograms as effective screening tools and are starting to cover some of the costs.

A great alternative for millennials and more

More importantly, thermography is becoming an excellent screening tool for younger women, screening years ahead of what mammograms typically show without any radiation.

A typical breast scan takes about 20 to 30 minutes, including the intake time required to capture a client's history. Results are given back to the client within two to three days after being read by a trained doctor.

Other benefits include:

- Thermography can be performed daily without any adverse effects.

- Thermography may be used monthly to assess the response of breast cancer treatment.

Here is how Mathews describes thermography:

"Thermography is a painless, non-invasive clinical test without any exposure to radiation. It is also known as DITI, Digital Infrared Thermal Imaging.

It is not a stand-alone tool but can be useful for earlier detection of breast disease than has been possible through self-breast exams, doctor's exams, and mammography alone.

The efficacy of thermography relies on clients having thermograms on a regular basis, usually once a year after a baseline has been established, to alert doctors to changes that can indicate early-stage breast disease."

The American College of Clinical Thermatology states:

"By performing thermography years before conventional mammography, a selected patient population at risk can be monitored more carefully, and then by accurately utilizing mammography or ultrasound as soon as is possible to detect the actual lesion (once it has grown large enough and dense enough to be seen on mammographic film), can increase the patient's treatment options and ultimately improve the outcome.

Thermographic breast scans are appropriate for all women. They are particularly useful for younger women ages 30-50 who have been told they have dense breast tissue, have a strong family history, have fibrocystic or cystic breasts, or for women who for many reasons can't undergo a mammogram.

One type of breast cancer, inflammatory, cannot be diagnosed with mammography as there is no 'lump' or tumor. This type is most commonly seen in younger women.

Mammograms look at the anatomical changes in the breast as they detect masses or lumps in the breast tissue. Thermograms look at vascular changes in the breast, as they detect blood flow patterns, inflammation, and asymmetries. The two detection methods complement each other and provide a holistic approach to early detection. With a multi-modal approach, a woman's chances for early breast cancer detection can be up to 95 percent."

Mathews suggests that it is important to have the first two breast scans done within a three-to-four month time period. Each person's thermal patterns are different depending on density of the breast tissue, fibrocystic changes, calcifications, cysts, etc. Active cancers double in size and heat in approximately 100 days. If there are any heat pattern changes and/or vascular changes from the first to the second scan, additional modalities will be requested by the doctors who interpret the images. If there are no changes, annual thermal scans are appropriate.

I had my first thermogram performed by Mathews on March 3, 2017, which was nearly five years after first being diagnosed with breast cancer on my right breast. The process was casual and relaxed, with Mathews greeting me with a hug and smile, then bringing me to a tiny room at an integrative health practice. The nurturing component she offered was so important to me after being in so many cold, sterile clinical environments in the past.

"Nurturing care explains why many patients often experience remarkable results when treated by complementary and alternative medicine (CAM) treatments, which include such therapies as acupuncture, Chinese medicine, homeopathy, Reiki, herbal medicine, energy medicine, craniosacral therapy, chiropractic medicine, and other modalities."

—Lissa Rankin, M.D., author of *New York Times* best-selling book, *Mind Over Medicine*

After capturing my medical history, and listening with compassion about my fears, Mathews then asked me to do the following:

Take off my clothes from the waist up, stand in front of a wall, with arms over head, looking straight ahead; then do the same turning to the left, turning to the right, then facing the wall with hands over hips. It took less than ten minutes, and I was later able to see on Mathews' computer screen the exact images she was viewing—although I needed a doctor to confirm the reading of report which is sent by email, regular mail, or as an electronic file.

I received my results via email two days later: "No suspicions" and "low risk" to both left and right breasts. Given my prior history with breast cancer, it was recommended I be tested again in three months to confirm my new baseline.

Elated by the test results, I also felt excited to have added Mathews as a new member to my health team. She honored my unique health journey, and offered confirmation of witnessing many other women successfully thrive using alternative routes as well.

She believes thermography and mammography can complement one another, having had experience with both.

It is important to note, Pam Mathews is also a trained Radiologic Technologist. She worked post-graduation at Johns Hopkins Hospital before moving to Massachusetts, where she worked at a high-risk-pregnancy hospital helping with pelvimetry exams and x-raying preemie babies on an on-call basis.

After nursing her last baby, she underwent several surgeries to remove calcified mammary glands and implant replacements because of scar tissue issues. Not knowing how much scatter radiation she had in her body, she did not want to have the mammograms the doctors were prescribing before each surgery and the compression was very painful.

Finding thermography was a godsend for her. She said it was a painless, non-radiation emitting, affordable diagnostic tool with no compression. With her experiences in mammography and thermography, she truly believes they are both valuable tools for being proactive about wellness and taking steps to prevent and identify disease at its earliest stages.

For further information visit:
spectrumthermography.com

EPILOGUE

A private victory

No one but me will truly know the depth of healing I did on myself to get the two clear body scans. My celebration of honoring my gut—and not doing unnecessary procedures and treatments—is such a silent victory.

Being a pioneer in using "energy as medicine" for five years, when so few would claim it as an adequate health tool, took great courage. I continue to lead groups, using the latest in neuroscience and the power of the collective unconscious, so together participants can elevate their minds and bodies for optimal healing and other life dreams.

Sitting alone with God, I *know* together we healed my body by courageously listening to its innate wisdom when so many discouraged me from going the natural path and trusting my gut. Stopping, pausing, and listening for divine guidance in this frenzied, action-based world takes stamina.

I wish I had a sign from above of "job well done" or a hug of comfort for all the tenacity it took to veer to the path of truth. *God, can we celebrate together? Is there some profound manifestation of our connection that I can share with the world? Please reveal the answer to me.*

I am also in awe of the women and men far braver than me, with later-stage diseases who had many more physical challenges than I have had to endure. Yet, my *calling* is to share ways I learned to live from love and worthiness. To do so, I've had to address the inner demons (beliefs) of past conditioning that kept me

204

operating at high stress levels, which I believe contributed to getting cancer.

Learning to train my mind for new possibilities
was nearly a full-time job!

The ending of this book is not just the completion of my deep entry into alternative models of healing; it is the ending of life as I knew it. I am leaving behind years of living in survival mode, trying too hard to be seen, known, acknowledged, and loved. Those external drivers never truly filled me up. Rather, they left me feeling empty and isolated.

There is no grasping left in me. That life of reaching exhausted me and my body.

These are some of my hard-earned lessons:

- I'm no longer willing to hold in the hurts of others' misdirected anger. I now set boundaries to protect my health. Being a doormat where others took advantage of my kindness and sensitivity no longer serves me. Speaking up to honor my needs and desires is something that protects me from getting ill again.

- I'm no longer willing to beg for help or be shamed by the debt I incurred based on past mistakes and the commitment I made to make my mind and body well—and serve this calling to bring my message to the masses. If others cannot find compassion within themselves to honor the courageous journey upon which I embarked, they don't meet the criteria to be included in my inner circle of support. It's not about the money; it's about empathy. Facing mortality is a life-altering event, and those who cannot hold and honor me with love and care, lack the type of courage it has taken me to claim *life*.

- I'm no longer willing to live as a victim. I chose life, to take enormous risks to live with no regret, and take big risks, like moving cross-country and reinventing my business and myself. I can easily claim these words I want to be remembered by: 'SHE CHOSE LIFE!' Hopefully, in the process, I have served others.

- I'm no longer willing to think I am less than, unworthy, or inadequate because a disease caused by stressors far beyond my control challenged me.

- I'm no longer willing to be shamed by the scar on my right breast, thinking I'm less than feminine because I don't have a perfect body.

On the five-year anniversary of my breast cancer diagnosis, I am sharing the truth about having endured a scary health threat. I live from a deeper sense of love for self and others, but I am no longer willing to "be nice" to placate others. Being authentic, and expressing who I truly am and what I feel, is more important for my health. Sometimes, I am looked at as "the bad guy" for doing so. Then, I remember wise words once uttered to me during my early stages of rebuilding my self-esteem years ago: "If one of us has to be uncomfortable, it does not have to be me."

Recreating oneself is sometimes messy. There are missteps and misunderstandings. Then, there are familiar faces from the past who do not know the new me. But how could they? I am just discovering her myself.

At the same time, I have the richest, most authentic relationships of my life with quality people from a diversity of backgrounds from the East to the West coast. Being an empath, I now understand how crucial it is to my health to be around those who can celebrate me. Reciprocity is a big word for me, too, and I hope to spend more time living and loving from it.

It seems rather paradoxical now that the tenacious *will* that served me in moving beyond a challenging childhood is the very *will* I have had to let go of now to surrender to a greater life than the one I tried to create.

I have come to the end of my "self," and have fully opened to God's plan for my life. Part of that plan is building a teaching platform around worthiness, and writing the sequel of my spiritual journey, *Bottoms Up... A Journey of Faith, Love and Conviction.*

I've kept brave decisions to myself so my children could prosper and embrace full lives as young adults without worrying about me, as I had done for my parents most of my life, taking on adult responsibilities as a child that should have never been mine.

The truth is, once you hear the "C" word, you are never the same again. I have chosen to take that word and make my life and me better. And yet "better" hasn't quite looked like what I expected, as I needed to let go of so many things to step into this life I am destined to live, from a whole new set of intentions and beliefs.

This journey is not for the faint-of-heart, but I can guarantee you that the faith acquired along the way created a spiritual wealth that can never be taken away.

I trust I am being guided to serve you in bigger ways than I ever imagined.

Stay posted.

In surrender to unlimited possibilities,

Gail

ABOUT THE AUTHOR

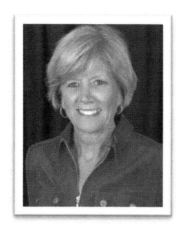

With the tools of an intuitive coach, the soul of a writer, and the wisdom of a reflective life, Gail Kauranen Jones brings a depth of expertise to her business, SupportMatters.com.

She has worked as a journalist, public relations executive, and content marketer before becoming an author, transformational coach, and wellness pioneer. She is also a blogger, frequently contributing to Arianna Huffington's Thrive Global along with many other venues such as The Wellness Universe.

In 2004, she published *To Hell and Back... Healing Your Way Through Transition* to help readers through four major transitions: career change, becoming a mother, caretaking elderly parents, and coping with the death of a loved one. Two years later, Gail's book was referenced as a great transition resource in Cheryl Richardson's *New York Times* best-selling book, *The Unmistakable Touch of Grace.*

Cancer as a Love Story: Developing the Mindset for Living came as a calling in the middle of the night as whispers in her mind. Gail then began her own deep "life pause" where she learned an extensive array of tools that guide her now in teaching the healing power of love and worthiness.

Gail lives in Phoenix, Arizona, where she facilitates leading-edge guided meditation groups. She blends the latest findings in neuroscience and "energy as medicine" with her unique coaching expertise.

It is her dream to keep expanding her speaking and group coaching platforms, having learned those who participate in a mind-body program can live more than two times longer and accelerate healing. She strongly believes in the power of the collective unconscious to help clients reach many other types of goals and dreams, in addition to improved health.

For more information about her book visit:
cancerasalovestory.com

"The pause—sometimes initiated by a life curveball like cancer or another one of the soul's promptings for redirecting life—is often the sacred place of becoming who we truly are."